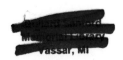

Mayo Clinic on Healthy Aging

Edward T. Creagan, M.D.

Editor-in-Chief

MASON CREST PUBLISHERS

Philadelphia, Pennsylvania

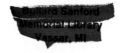

Mayo Clinic on Healthy Aging provides reliable, practical, easy-to-understand information on preparing for and dealing with the aging process. Much of this information comes directly from the experience of physicians and administrative specialists at Mayo Clinic. Personal stories in this book are composites representative of experiences seen by Mayo Clinic physicians. This book supplements the advice of your physician, whom you should consult for individual medical problems. *Mayo Clinic on Healthy Aging* does not endorse any company or product. MAYO, MAYO CLINIC, MAYO CLINIC HEALTH INFORMATION and the Mayo triple-shield logo are marks of Mayo Foundation for Medical Education and Research.

Hardcover Library Edition Published 2002
Mason Crest Publishers
370 Reed Road
Suite 302
Broomall, PA 19008-0914
(866) MCP-BOOK (toll free)

First printing

1 2 3 4 5 6 7 8 9 10

Library of Congress Cataloging-in-Publication Data on file at the Library of Congress

ISBN 1-59084-224-3

Printed in the United States of America

About Healthy Aging

Healthy aging doesn't occur by accident. It's not a chance event, governed by your genes and circumstances. Healthy aging requires thoughtful, careful planning and a commitment to a lifestyle focused on such things as proper nutrition, regular physical, spiritual and social activity and adequate financial resources. Individuals who age best are people who are positive minded, proactive in their decision making and well informed. They are realistic. They know that gains in wisdom may be associated with losses in physical ability.

Within these pages you'll find advice you can use to successfully manage the aging process and maintain or improve the quality of your living. This book is based on the expertise of Mayo Clinic doctors and the advice they give day in and day out in caring for their patients. Mayo chaplains and administrative specialists helped with the chapters on spirituality and finances.

About Mayo Clinic

Mayo Clinic evolved from the frontier practice of Dr. William Worrall Mayo, and the partnership of his two sons, William J. and Charles J. Mayo, in the early 1900s. Pressed by the demands of their busy surgical practice in Rochester, Minn., the Mayo brothers invited other physicians to join them, pioneering the private group practice of medicine. Today, with more than 2,000 physicians and scientists at its three major locations in Rochester, Minn., Jacksonville, Fla., and Scottsdale, Ariz., Mayo Clinic is dedicated to providing comprehensive diagnosis, accurate answers and effective treatments and to being a dependable source of health information for patients and the public.

With its depth of knowledge, experience and expertise, Mayo Clinic occupies an unparalleled position as a health information resource. Since 1983, Mayo Clinic has published reliable health information for millions of consumers through award-winning newsletters, books and online services. Revenue from the publishing activities supports Mayo Clinic programs, including medical education and research.

Editorial staff

Editor in chief
Edward T. Creagan, M.D.

Managing editor
David E. Swanson

Copy editor
Mary Duerson

Editorial researchers
Deirdre A. Herman
Michelle K. Hewlett

Contributing writers
Howard E. Bell
Linda Kephart Flynn
Michael J. Flynn

D. R. Martin
Stephen M. Miller
Robin Silverman
Susan Wichmann

Creative director
Daniel W. Brevick

Layout and production artist
Craig R. King

Editorial assistant
Carol A. Olson

Indexer
Larry Harrison

Reviewers and additional contributors

Kim M. Anderson, C.F.P.
Rev. Warren D. Anderson,
   M.Div.
Carolyn S. Beck, Ph.D.
M. Kim Bryan, J.D., C.F.P.
Rev. Jane H. Chelf, M.Div., R.N.
Darryl S. Chutka, M.D.
Richard C. Edwards
Andrew E. Good, M.D.
Marita Heller
Edward R. Laskowski, M.D.
Roger A. Lindahl

Rev. Dean V. Marek
Paul S. Mueller, M.D.
Leon D. Rabe
Teresa A. Rummans, M.D.
Yogesh Shah, M.D.
Ray W. Squires, Ph.D.
Michael J. Stuart, M.D.
Jeffrey M. Thompson, M.D.
Marchant Woodhouse Van
   Gerpen, M.D.
Janet L. Vittone, M.D.

Preface

We are in one of the greatest migrations in the history of the civilized world. Approximately 78 million so-called baby boomers, individuals born in the United States after the end of World War II, are marching into their post-employment years. If you're one of them, this book is for you.

About 100 years ago, the average individual lived fewer than 50 years. If you were born in the 1940s, you can expect to enjoy a productive, creative life into your 70s or 80s. The 85-plus group is the fastest-growing segment of the population in this country. As the famous ragtime pianist Eubie Blake said on his 100th birthday "If I'd known I was gonna live this long, I'd have taken better care of myself."

Taking better care of yourself physically, emotionally, socially, spiritually and financially is what this book is about. The opportunities you have to reframe your life in your post-employment years may be lost in the absence of effective planning and preparation. Never before has a deliberate, proactive approach to aging been of such vital importance to the quality of a person's life in what for many people will be the most exciting adventure of all — the final decades.

The information in this book will enable you to make informed choices about issues that matter as you, and those you love, sift through the bewildering maze of information and misinformation that's available on healthy aging. You'll also find stories about people who've made a few miscalculations along the way — and helpful tips on how you can learn from their experiences.

Edward T. Creagan, M.D.
Editor in chief

Contents

Chapter 1

Facts and phases

Take-home messages

- Assume you'll live a very long time.
- Your senior years can be your best years.
- Plan now for your final decade of life.

If you're over 40, you've undoubtedly confronted some facts about growing older. You've probably peered into the mirror at a face that has developed a few more wrinkles. Or you've noticed that aches and pains linger longer after you've played one too many rounds of golf. Most likely you've found yourself planning how much more money you need to stash away each month to ensure a comfortable retirement.

Until we're in our fourth or fifth decade, aging rarely means much to us, even though it's a lifelong process that begins the moment we are born. Childhood, adolescence and young adulthood are filled with beliefs of immortality. It's only when we notice physical changes in ourselves that we accept that we actually may be getting older. Only when we start to see our parents and friends aging — and sometimes dying — do we begin to see the possibility of our own personal end.

If you're more than 60, you've probably already encountered the realities of aging, but also may have realized that you have a lot more life left than you'd once thought. Perhaps you're taking care of parents in their 80s who never, in their wildest dreams, expected such longevity. Maybe you're about to retire and haven't a clue what to do with the extra time you'll have — or you're worried that the blissful days you plan to spend traveling or golfing may not be enough to really satisfy you.

Whatever your life stage, aging, as they say, sure beats the alternative. But you now have countless ways to do more than just grow older. You can, in fact, make your older years the best time of your life. It may mean altering your behavior or changing a few deep-seated attitudes, but you do have choices about how you age. As the famous ragtime pianist Eubie Blake said on his 100th birthday, "If I'd known I was gonna live this long, I'd have taken better care of myself."

How long will you live?

| Year | Life expectancy at birth | | Additional years after 65 | |
	Male	Female	Male	Female
1900	46.4	49.0	11.4	11.7
1920	54.5	56.3	11.8	12.3
1940	61.4	65.7	11.9	13.4
1960	66.7	73.2	12.9	15.9
1980	69.9	77.5	14.0	18.4
2000	73.2	79.7	15.8	19.3

Timing, as they say, is everything. If you were a baby in 1900 you could expect to reach your mid- to late 40s. If you survived the onslaught of childhood diseases and you reached 65, you'd probably live until your mid-70s. On the other hand, if you were born last year and you live to age 65, you can expect to live until your early to mid-80s.

Source: Office of the Chief Actuary, Social Security Administration

What is aging anyway?

The realities of aging have changed, even though some of our beliefs about it have not. Retiring at 65, for example, used to mean that you were near the end of your life. When Social Security was launched in 1935, life expectancy was about 63. Politicians figured there would be plenty of able-bodied workers to support the few people who actually made it to the designated age — and that those who did get a monthly check wouldn't last long anyway. These days, however, increased life expectancies mean that most retirees will receive Social Security benefits for about two decades. In other words, 65-year-olds aren't even close to being old yet.

In the last century, improvements in medicine, science and technology have helped us all to live longer, healthier lives. Between 1900 and 2000, average life expectancy at birth rose from about 47 years to 76, a 62 percent increase in our allotted time on the planet.

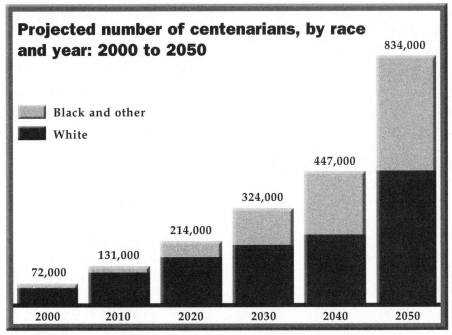

Projected number of centenarians, by race and year: 2000 to 2050

Black and other
White

2000: 72,000
2010: 131,000
2020: 214,000
2030: 324,000
2040: 447,000
2050: 834,000

Source: J.C. Day, 1996, *Population Projections of the United States by Age, Sex, Race, and Hispanic Origin*. U.S. Bureau of Census, Current Population Reports, P25-1130, U.S. Government Printing Office, Washington, D.C.

And it gets even better if you can live through childhood ailments, infections, cancer and heart disease. For example, a woman who reaches her 50th birthday today, with no cancer or heart disease, can expect to see 92. The average healthy woman who is 65 today can expect to live to 84.

Of all the people who have ever lived to be 65, half are currently alive. Moreover, the 85-plus group is the fastest growing demographic segment in the United States, although the number of centenarians has exploded as well. Between 2000 and 2050, 100-year-olds will increase in number by nearly 1,100 percent to a record 834,000 people.

In the last 10 years, scientists made great progress in the battle against aging. Currently, more than 100,000 research projects to slow

An iron in the fire

My parents told me if I worked hard and gave 110 percent, my employer would take care of me. For a while that's how it was, but that changed in ways I never dreamed it could.

For many years, I came to work early and stayed late. I went the extra mile for clients, making follow-up calls and personal visits to make sure our product arrived on time and the customer was happy. Back at the office, I was good at navigating choppy political waters. I quickly rose to middle management. I was a survivor. I was comfortable and figured I'd be there until I retired. Boy was I wrong.

Early warnings crossed my desk in the form of memos about the "need for cost containment" and "efficiencies of outsourcing." Custodial services, food services, security — one by one whole departments were outsourced. The new MBA hired guns roaming the halls were young and had no sense of loyalty or connection to the rest of us.

Then it hit me — that's the point. This is how they show us older employees the door. Replace us with youngsters, pay them lower wages and fewer benefits, and save a bundle. In the corporation's eyes I was obsolete — a liability, not an asset. I knew then I needed a new plan.

I took stock of my interests and talents. I like people and I'm an avid reader and book lover. I often day dreamed about volunteering aging are under way in numerous disciplines throughout the world. Scientists are studying everything from cloning for spare parts to how DNA mutations affect aging to fighting cancer with viruses.

Clearly, old isn't what it used to be. And as 78 million baby boomers approach their retirement years, the definition will continue to evolve. The United Nations expects that by 2050 nearly 2 billion people will be at least 60 — a number equal to the current combined populations of North America, Europe and India. Experts talk about what a giant influx of new retirees will do to America's Social Security system, but everything else will be affected, too, from health care to families, from employment to real estate prices.

at the library after I retired. Would they actually pay me to do what I love?

I met with the county library supervisor and told her I'd be leaving my profession in a couple years, maybe sooner. She explained that library jobs don't open often. When they do, many people apply and there's a formal hiring process to ensure fairness. So I left her my résumé, then made a point to check in with her every few months in a friendly, nonpushy way so she could get to know me and see I was really interested. Just knowing I had another iron in the fire made work more bearable.

Two years after that first interview, my persistence paid off. The county library system posted a job opening for an assistant librarian in my little town. I applied and got the job even though I was in my early 50s. Life is good again.

Manufacturing manager — Alexander, Ohio

Points to ponder

- Retirement may come sooner than you think. Plan ahead.
- Inventory your interests and talents. Be assertive in finding ways to use them.
- Be prepared to reinvent yourself.
- Develop a toolbox of skills and contacts that are portable. If the corporate ship sinks, your career will sail on.

More in the middle

A longer life might not be desirable if the additional years were simply tacked on at the end, when declining health becomes more of a possibility. But it appears, instead, that we're spending more time in the middle. Already, social scientists have coined a word for these extra years. "Middlescence," they say, is akin to adolescence, which also defines a group not quite ready for the next stage in life.

Middlescence runs from about 40 to 60, a stage people once considered middle age. Now it's often a period of growth and renewal, when it's still possible to embark on adventures once reserved for those much younger. Consider, for example, the birthrate among women over 40 in the United States, which has increased by 50 percent in the last two decades. Deferring childbirth for 10 to 20 years

Differences between the sexes

It's a simple fact that women live longer than men. In most developed countries, women can expect to outlive men by about 7 years, although the difference is even greater in some nations, such as Russia. In the United States, nearly half of all women over 65 are widows.

Is it biological? Gerontologists think not. Instead, they say, it comes down to a lifetime of behaviors. Researchers acknowledge that men could avoid as much as 70 percent of the illnesses they grapple with by getting regular checkups and by taking better care of themselves.

What do women do that men don't do? Women are more likely to watch their diets, exercise, seek out medical opinions, buy self-help books and join a health club. They also go in for lifesaving health screenings far more often than men. In addition, men are socialized to tough it out, and they often feel self-conscious when they complain about their aches and pains.

When it comes to life expectancies, men lag far behind in the battle of the sexes. Medical researchers, however, have obviously shown that it doesn't have to be that way.

"may be the most radical voluntary alteration of the life cycle," wrote Gail Sheehy in her 1995 book, *New Passages.*

But added years also mean that some of us may spend more time in an incapacitated state at the end of our lives, in part because the nation has done too little to promote healthy aging. And that is where this book comes in. A century ago, the average adult was ill for only 1 percent of his or her life; today's average adult will spend more than 10 percent of his or her life dealing with illness. Medical advances have eliminated many of the diseases that once felled people in their youth, but science has failed to adequately address chronic conditions that accompany aging. And even though we're taking better care of ourselves as a group, the rates of obesity, sedentary lifestyle, smoking and alcohol abuse are still too high.

It's not about retirement

You're not suddenly "old" when you hit 65, become a grandparent or go through menopause. You're old only when you think you are, when you "accept an attitude of dormancy, dependence on others, a substantial limitation on your physical and mental activity, and restrictions on the number of other people with whom you interact," wrote former president Jimmy Carter in his 1998 book, *The Virtues of Aging.*

In other words, aging is largely in your head. Well, almost largely in your head. Read on. While your body may age, your mind, for the most part, will stay as young as you feel. If you expect to live a long life filled with physical vitality, humor and social connectedness, then that fundamental belief becomes an internal diagram that to a large degree will predict your future. But if you're convinced that old age will be a time of emptiness, depression and sickness, you'll probably find yourself experiencing a mental desolation that will certainly lead to physical debilitation. In general, your negative expectations will make you age faster than nature intended.

Everything counts

Of course, it's not just what's in your mind when you hit a particular birthday. Your quality of life in old age will be an accumulation of the habits, beliefs, experiences and attitudes you've collected as you go through life. Do you believe, for example, that exercise is good for you? Do you act on that by walking 30 minutes every day? Then you'll probably be healthier at 70 than someone who considers exercise a waste of time. Are you a person who views minor setbacks as a personal challenge, or do you think failure is a conspiracy against you? Studies show that many more optimists than pessimists live to a ripe old age.

In fact, the Centers for Disease Control and Prevention estimates that more than half of your potential for lifelong health will be determined by your own attitudes and actions. In addition to your attitudes about exercise and failure, consider these questions: Do you smoke or chew tobacco? Do you drink alcohol excessively? Are you carrying too many pounds? Your quality of life in old age can even come down to such seemingly benign actions as whether you wear sunscreen or seat belts. In the end, it all adds up.

A world of possibilities

If you were a baby girl in 1940, you could expect to live until you were about 66 (if you were a boy, about 61). But life spans have changed, and now you may be 70 or older and feeling just fine. During your youth, you didn't think much about retirement because your parents probably didn't retire. In those days, you worked until you died, and that was about it. At the turn of the 20th century, nearly 90 percent of older men who were able to work did so, compared with fewer than 20 percent of older men who work today. Older men and women who work today generally work because they want to.

Indeed, these children of the 1940s have been at the forefront of an aging population that has had to invent a new reality for themselves in old age, one that includes considerable free time after retirement. What have they done? Some have started new businesses; others have embarked on graduate degrees. Some have taken up new hobbies, learned to use the computer or traveled the world. Still others have done volunteer service or spent time caring for their grandchildren.

For the most part, however, they've had to figure it all out on their own. Although medical researchers have been busy devising solutions to life-threatening illnesses, no one was working on a worthwhile idea for what these countless mature men and women might do with all the additional years they've been given. That could be why many retirees find themselves searching for meaningful activities, and why some 40 million of them spend an average of 43 hours a week watching television.

Something to do

The activities designed for older people will almost certainly continue to grow as the oldest of the baby boomers start turning 65 in 2011. Just as their sheer numbers have inspired everything from youth programs to products that smooth facial wrinkles, their advancing years can open new opportunities for volunteering, travel and education.

But don't think you'll simply be able to wait for your next assignment. Even if you're offered newly organized programs — along the lines of the Senior Corps, for example, which galvanizes some 500,000 people who work part time as foster grandparents, caregivers, tutors and more (see its Web site at *www.seniorcorps.org*) — you'll still have decisions to make about how you want to spend your later years. You are in the driver's seat. But no one will start the engine for you.

What you decide will be incredibly important. After all, your primary purpose shouldn't be just to stay alive as long as you can, but to savor every opportunity for joy, productivity and fulfillment. The later years can be a time of renewal, when it's possible to explore options and prospects, especially if you have the gift of good health. You may find yourself freed from some responsibilities, such as child rearing, or taking on new ones, such as caring for your parents. What you do with your circumstances will, of course, be yours to determine.

What are your prospects?

The big question about how you will age centers on your health. If you're a healthy 65- or 70-year-old, an abundance of lifestyle choices will lie waiting at your feet as you grow older. If you're disabled you'll be limited in what you can do with your older years.

Surprisingly, genes account for only about one-third of the effects of aging; the rest are mainly due to lifestyle and environment. If your father and grandfather both died young from heart attacks, for example, you may be inclined to believe the same fate awaits you. Although you may have a genetic tendency for heart disease, diet, exercise, medications and avoiding tobacco play a significant role in whether you actually develop a heart condition. This means that you have some control over how you age. Your mind and emotions are important.

A fellow traveler

When I joined the force I found the work exhilarating. But by age 56, I'd had enough of gangs, drugs and violence. I woke up to my own mortality and no longer wanted to be a human target for society's fringe performers.

After 6 months of early retirement, I was going wacko with boredom. I gained 20 pounds and, I kid you not, had a callous on my remote control finger. I still had my commercial driver's license, something I got on a whim a few years ago. So I had that renewed and got a job driving a cement truck. That was OK for a couple months, but it was seasonal. I saw an ad in the newspaper for a tour bus driver, so I applied and got it. Who'd have thought I would enjoy it so much.

My job was to drive retirees to casinos, shopping centers, museums and other touristy places. After a couple of weeks, I started recognizing familiar faces. I don't know if it's because I'm a good listener or because there's something about being a bus driver that makes people want to tell you their stories.

Passengers knew I stayed on the bus, sometimes for hours,

It all adds up

It can't be stated too strongly: Your youthful and middle age habits will follow you into old age. Years of cigarette smoking, excessive alcohol use, too little exercise and overeating do physical damage that is often wrongly attributed to age. A recent study by Stanford University researchers found that middle-aged people who watched their weight, exercised and didn't smoke not only lived longer but had fewer years of sickness and less dependence on others as they grew older.

Can you undo a lifetime of bad habits? Researchers say it's never too late to clean up your act. Take cigarettes, for example. If you quit smoking, your risk of heart disease begins to fall almost immediately. Within five years, you won't be much more likely to have heart disease than someone who never smoked. It'll take 15 years to reduce your chances for lung disease, but you'll never diminish your odds if you don't quit.

while everyone was off doing stuff, so they'd come out and talk about divorces, bankruptcies, successes, failures, health problems, adult kids who didn't turn out so well — all of it. We had a lot of laughs, too. More than a few folks said hanging out on the bus was more fun than slot machines. And a lot less expensive.

What the passengers maybe didn't know is I was having as much fun as they were. I became a "psychiatrist" for the 44 passengers. I never doled out advice about stuff I didn't know anything about. I was just a port in the storm, someone to talk to. I never felt so needed.

Correctional officer — Detroit, Mich.

Points to ponder

- Find occupations, hobbies and volunteer opportunities that make you feel good about yourself.

- Be creative and open-minded about trying new experiences. They may open up a new chapter in your life.

- Stay connected with family, friends and groups.

As for exercise, studies have shown that even frail nursing home residents on strength-training regimens will achieve more than stronger biceps. Their overall health and ability to perform activities of daily living improve as well. But when the strength training is stopped, the beneficial improvements are lost. So strength or resistance training needs to be part of a complete exercise program.

Get started now

No matter what your age, you can — and should — begin preparing now for your later years. If you're a middlescent, you've got plenty of time to gear up for your old age, whether it's initiating an exercise program, devising a better diet or fine-tuning your social skills. If you're already retired, it's not too late to decide how — and how well — you want to live for the next 10 or 20 or 30 years. Maybe you want to learn and travel through the Elderhostel program or educate yourself about computers on www.seniornet.org or volunteer at your local school or attend church every Sunday. You are the master of your own quality of life. You are the captain of your ship.

Within these pages, we will provide you the tools, tactics and strategies to make your older years meaningful, productive and creative. We'll help you answer questions such as these:

- What will keep you healthy?
- Who will make a difference in your life?
- How can you keep your independence?

We've gathered the latest information on aging from our seasoned experts to give you a big picture view of a most important topic.

What you'll learn

In a nutshell, we'll give you tips for healthy aging that include ideas like these:

Exercise your mind. Give up any expectations about your brain cells dying as you reach old age. Research shows that actively engaged people are more likely to remain mentally and physically stimulated and, as a result, to enjoy a better quality of life. Be open to new opportunities for learning.

Keep physically active. If you're a sedentary 80-year-old, you could use half your physical stamina just taking a shower. But you can avoid that scenario with regular exercise. In fact, exercise is probably the single most important thing you can do to age successfully. Physical fitness will allow you to function better in everyday life — and live longer and stronger even in the face of other health problems or bad habits. You don't have to join the local heath club to keep physically active. Look for daily opportunities to be more physically active. Walking, swimming and cycling are easy on your joints.

Eat well. Mom was right. Including plenty of fruits, vegetables and whole grains in your diet not only is good for you but will lead to a longer life. So will limiting saturated fats, cholesterol, sugar and sodium in your diet. A diet for successful aging will also include plenty of water.

Eliminate bad habits. You can't abolish every risk from your life, but you do have control over some things that are bad for you. In particular, if you want to live a long and healthy life, avoid excessive alcohol and nicotine in all its forms, including cigarettes, secondhand smoke and chewing tobacco.

Watch your attitude. You are what you think. Throughout your life, it's important to stay focused on what's important and to shrug off what isn't. An ability to roll with the punches and a sense of humor are tools that can help you cope. Needless worries sap energy and vitality. As speaker and author Loretta LaRoche writes in her 1998 book, *Relax: You May Only Have a Few Minutes Left*, "No one ever said on his deathbed, 'I wish I hadn't laughed so much.'"

Nurture your spirit. Have faith. No matter what you call your source of inspiration, it's important to define and practice your spirituality. Research shows that people who rely on prayer have an easier time getting through life's difficult periods, and the people you get to know in a faith community will sustain you, too.

Stay connected. Being part of a social network of friends and family is one of the best predictors of longevity. How important is it? In America, people 75 or older who live alone have more than twice the mortality rate of those with companions. You can also stay connected by volunteering or joining a support group. Nurture relationships with younger friends. Younger friends provide enthusiasm; older adults provide wisdom.

Plan ahead. Whatever you do, you will age — or at least that's the hope. But you can determine for yourself some aspects of how that process will happen. Think about your financial affairs, your future living arrangements and how you've provided for loved ones. Make sure you've defined what's important to you now and what will become more critical as you move through the years. You don't have to be rich to be happy, but try to budget for activities and a lifestyle that you value.

Sure, it's important to be certain your 401(k) is fully funded, but also think about how and with whom you want to spend your time, what kind of life you want to lead and what kind of person you want to be. As you know, you won't suddenly arrive at old age: It will be merely an extension of who you are now, what happens to you along the way, and whatever changes you make to improve your life. As you read this book and reflect on the need for adjustments in the way you live, remember that your later years can be the richest time of your life, if you want them to be. The choice — for the most part — is up to you.

Chapter 2

Your body

- Know how aging affects your body.
- You have the power to deal with declines.
- Take action to maintain your health.

What can you expect from your body as you get older? Wouldn't it be nice if your doctor could hand you a memo outlining all of the changes to come? But we each respond to the march of time in a unique fashion, influenced by our genes, our lifestyle choices, our environment and a multitude of other factors.

Dealing with change

No one can predict how long you will live. But we all have a few things in common. As Dr. Charles H. Mayo once observed, "The only thing that is permanent is change." Our flesh, bones, muscles, nerves and organs have a limited life span. Some parts tend to lose their shine or wear out sooner than others do. Others, if cared for properly, seem to weather the years more gracefully.

This chapter describes some of the ways in which your organs and body systems change as you age, as well as some diseases and disorders that are more common among older adults. Not all of these changes and diseases are inevitable. Much of the decline we blame on aging is actually due to inactivity and other lifestyle choices.

This chapter also provides information to help you prevent, minimize or at least cope with many of these changes. The final section, called "Preserving your lifestyle," includes tips on fitness, nutrition, sexuality and sleep, to help you maintain or improve your quality of life as you age.

Your bones, muscles and joints

Although you might think of your bones as hard, rigid and unchanging, they constantly undergo renewal and respond to the demands placed on them. Your bones reach their maximal mass between ages 25 and 35. During the years that follow, they decline slightly in size and density. One consequence of this shrinkage is that your height may decrease. Another is that your bones become more brittle, making you prone to fractures.

Problems that affect your bones and joints tend to be chronic and often worsen over time. Most are not life-threatening, but they can cause you to alter your lifestyle significantly and lead to disability.

Muscles, tendons and joints generally lose some strength and flexibility as you age. If you have led an active life, by age 60 your muscles will have lost some of the strength they had in your youth. You will have less flexibility, your reflexes will be slower and your coordination will be poorer. You'll probably need to take a little more time getting to where you want to go.

If you have a disease that saps your energy or an ailment that affects your mobility, you may experience greater impairment. Arthritis and osteoporosis, for example, can slow you down considerably, particularly if you led a more sedentary lifestyle before these problems developed.

Arthritis. Most arthritis is simple deterioration of a joint. Heredity, diet, excessive weight and previous injuries and diseases in your joints are possible contributing factors. But so is everyday use.

Osteoarthritis, sometimes called degenerative arthritis or degenerative joint disease, is present to some degree in more than 80 percent of older adults. It usually causes pain and stiffness and starts in the spine or the large joints such as your hips and knees, which bear the weight of your body. It can also show up elsewhere, such as in the knuckles. Because your natural response to a painful joint is to move it less, you use the muscles in the area less frequently and they start to shrink and lose strength.

Rheumatoid arthritis is an autoimmune disease, a disease in which your body's immune system attacks itself. In most cases rheumatoid arthritis, which is much less common than osteoarthritis, affects joints in your wrists, hands, feet and ankles. Affected joints are swollen, painful, tender and warm during the initial attack and during flare-ups that may follow. Although it is often chronic, rheumatoid arthritis tends to vary in severity and may come and go. The disease can strike at any age, but most often it develops in people ages 20 to 50. It affects roughly twice as many women as men.

Osteoporosis. Osteoporosis is caused by a gradual loss of mineral content from bones, making them thinner, weaker and more prone to fracture. Unlike other bone and joint problems, osteoporosis is symptom free at first. A bone fracture may be the first indication of a problem. Losing height also may be a sign.

About 25 million Americans have osteoporosis. The disease causes more than 1 million fractures every year in this country — usually in the spine, hip or wrist. Fractures from osteoporosis are about twice as common in women as in men. But by age 75, one-third of men have some osteoporosis.

Certain fractures, such as those of the hip, may severely limit or end your independence or even your life. Although surgery to repair the fracture is usually effective, the recovery period is lengthy, and life-threatening complications can occur. In fact, the death rate within 1 year of a hip fracture ranges from 12 percent to 20 percent.

What you can do

Rest, pain relievers and heat. Rest, pain relievers and heat usually help ease joint and muscle pain. Acetaminophen (Tylenol) and non-steroidal anti-inflammatory drugs, so-called NSAIDs (en-SAYDS), such as ibuprofen and naproxen, can be quite effective. If painful joints or muscles don't respond to these self-care measures, talk to your doctor. A newer generation of prescription pain relievers, called COX-2 inhibitors (Celebrex, Vioxx, Mobic), are now available. Injections or joint surgeries such as hip replacement may provide good recovery.

Two dietary supplements called glucosamine and chondroitin sulfate have gained a lot of attention as a treatment for osteoarthritis. Until more research data is available, Mayo Clinic physicians consider the supplements to be potentially useful for people with significant symptoms. As with any medication, consult your doctor before using these supplements.

Exercise regularly. Staying active is one of the best weapons against osteoporosis and loss of mobility due to arthritis. If you're in good physical condition before an accident or an illness, you'll recover more quickly. Weight-bearing activities, that is, any activity you do on your feet with your bones supporting your weight, and strength training help preserve and strengthen your bones. Water aerobics is easier on your joints. (See "Exercise," page 43.)

Maintain a healthy weight. Losing excess weight helps reduce stress and strain on your muscles and joints.

Consider hormone replacement therapy. If you're a woman, talk to your doctor about hormone replacement therapy (HRT) to prevent or treat osteoporosis. Estrogen, a component of hormone therapy, slows calcium loss, restores lost bone and reduces the risk of spine or hip fractures by at least 50 percent. It's most effective the first 6 to 8 years following menopause. But if you already have osteoporosis, starting HRT can still increase your bone density. If you can't or don't want to take estrogen, other prescription drugs can help slow bone loss and may increase bone density.

Get adequate calcium and vitamin D. Calcium and vitamin D are essential nutrients for building and sustaining bone mass. Dairy products, such as milk, yogurt and cheese, are rich in calcium. Liver, fish and egg yolks are rich in vitamin D. And just 15 minutes of sunshine at least three times a week helps your body make its own vitamin D.

Don't smoke. Smoking interferes with calcium absorption and decreases the amount of the hormone estrogen that your body produces. Estrogen helps protect against bone loss.

Limit alcohol. Excessive consumption of alcohol can reduce your rate of bone formation and may impair your body's ability to absorb calcium (see page 33).

Your brain and nervous system

Your brain needs a constant supply of oxygen and nutrients from blood delivered through several key arteries. One of the most important age-related changes that can affect your brain occurs in these arteries. Over time, fatty deposits may accumulate in your artery walls (atherosclerosis). These deposits may narrow the passageway through your vessels, putting you at risk of stroke.

Stroke. Most strokes occur when a blood clot blocks blood flow to the brain. If the blockage continues for more than a few minutes, brain cells in the affected area may be destroyed.

Stroke is our nation's third leading killer and the leading cause of serious disability. People who have had a previous stroke or experienced mild stroke symptoms that disappear within 24 hours (called a transient ischemic attack, or TIA) are at much greater risk of a stroke. Other risk factors include high blood pressure, heart disease, diabetes, smoking and a diet high in cholesterol and saturated fat. In general, men, blacks, people over 55 and people with a family history of stroke also are at higher risk.

What you can do

Learn the warning signs of stroke. Seek immediate medical attention if you notice one or more of these symptoms:

- Sudden numbness, weakness or paralysis in your face, an arm or a leg, usually on one side of your body
- Loss of speech, or trouble talking or understanding speech

- Sudden blurred or decreased vision, usually in one eye
- Dizziness, loss of balance or coordination
- A sudden, severe headache, with no apparent cause

Get your blood and your blood pressure checked. You may have high blood pressure without even knowing it. If your blood fats (lipids) are high, your doctor will recommend lifestyle changes and possibly a medication.

Quit smoking. Smokers have a 50 percent greater risk of having a stroke than nonsmokers do.

Cut back on fat and salt. Cutting back on fat and salt intake will help decrease your risk of high cholesterol, high blood pressure and obesity.

Stay active. Exercising can strengthen your heart, improve your circulation and lower your blood pressure and cholesterol levels. Check with your physician before beginning any new exercise program. (See "Exercise," page 43.)

If you drink alcohol do so in moderation. Consuming more than one or two drinks a day can raise your blood pressure (see page 33).

Dementia and Parkinson's disease

You were born with billions of brain cells. As you age, some of these cells may die or malfunction. Your body also gradually produces less of the chemicals that your brain cells need to work. In most cases you will not notice any change because surrounding cells can usually compensate for this loss. But when progressive deterioration occurs in any part of your nervous system, you gradually will lose some ability to function. This loss can impair coordination, mental ability, muscular movement and muscular control. Two disorders of the brain are dementia and Parkinson's disease.

Dementia. Dementia is a progressive decline in intellectual and social abilities that affects a person's daily functioning. Alzheimer's disease is the most common form of dementia. For more information about Alzheimer's disease, memory loss and age-related mental changes, see Chapter 3.

Parkinson's disease. Parkinson's disease typically occurs in people older than 50. More than 1 million Americans have the disorder. The hallmark of Parkinson's disease is tremors. The tremors can become so disruptive that you have difficulty holding a fork steady enough to eat or a newspaper still enough to read. Eventually, balance problems and muscle rigidity may be just as disabling.

The cause of Parkinson's remains unknown. Researchers do know that the disease occurs when nerve cells, called neurons, die or become impaired. Once affected, these neurons no longer produce a chemical called dopamine, which is necessary for smooth, purposeful muscle activity.

What you can do

A variety of medications are available to treat Parkinson's and slow its progression. The challenge is to find a medication that relieves symptoms with a minimum of side effects. In its advanced stages, Parkinson's usually requires medical or surgical treatment. But you can help improve your mobility, balance and coordination with muscle-stretching exercises and physical therapy. (See "Exercise," page 43.) There's preliminary evidence that coffee drinkers may have a lower risk of Parkinson's. Encouraging developments from research offer hope.

Diabetes

Diabetes mellitus is a chronic disease that affects the way your body uses digested food for energy and growth, resulting in abnormally high amounts of blood glucose (a form of sugar). Type 2 diabetes, also called adult-onset diabetes, usually develops after age 40. You're at risk of type 2 diabetes if you're physically inactive or overweight or if you have a family member with the disease.

If you have diabetes, your body does not produce or properly use insulin, a hormone needed to allow your tissues to properly use blood sugar (glucose). Left untreated, diabetes can cause a variety of life-threatening complications. Heart and blood vessel disease is the biggest of these, putting you at increased risk of heart attack, stroke, high blood pressure and circulation problems that could require amputation of toes or even limbs. Kidney failure, nerve damage and blindness can also occur.

A limb for a limb

I was slowing down by the time I hit my mid-50s. But I worked through the tiredness and grinding hours because good people counted on me.

I was a union negotiator and worked in the same tire factory my dad worked in for 40 years, after he came to this country from Sicily speaking hardly a word of English.

I've got the gift of gab, and I guess you could say I'm nobody's fool. I got along good with other guys on the shop floor. Some of them called me "the mouth," which I took as a compliment because that's how they meant it. Next thing I knew, they elected me our union representative at age 31.

Over the years, I hammered out some tough contracts with management. We won some really good concessions, especially for our health benefits and severance packages. I remember a 2-month stretch when I was in bitter brass knuckle negotiations for 10 or 12 hours a day.

Some nights I'd hop the red-eye back to New York and put in a full day arm-wrestling with the desk jockeys and bean counters back there. I was good at what I did, and everybody knew it. So even though I was feeling the years, I kept at it because I was the voice for so many good people. Little did I know that a stupid accident that had nothing to do with work would put me out to pasture.

A limb on our 80-year-old white oak rubbed against the side of the house. When it was windy, the branches scratched against the bedroom shutter and drove my wife nuts. It'd been doing that for about a year. Don't ask me why I decided to take care of the problem on a drizzly, windblown, 40-degree Saturday in early November. Maybe because it was a piece-of-cake job and one more thing I could check off my chore list. I was bulletproof. So I thought.

I'm up on the aluminum ladder. Branches are swaying in the wind. I've got the chain saw in my right hand and the #&!@%! limb to my left — a little too far to the left as it turned out. A little voice in my head said, "Hey dummy, get down off the ladder and move it." But I was cold and in a hurry. I reached with the saw. My foot slipped, and then things happened in slow motion as I fell from roof level.

I had the presence of mind to toss the chain saw as far as I could. I felt searing pain in my right arm and was horrified to see it bent at a 45-degree angle. A huge pool of blood was soaking through my pant leg. No, I didn't cut it with the saw. Wouldn't you know I hit the cement sidewalk instead of the grass and broke a blood vessel on impact. My arm, meanwhile, was busted in two places.

By the time my wife got home from the store, I was lying there pale. The paramedics got there in 10 minutes and took me to the hospital. Six weeks and two operations later, I was discharged. After 4 weeks of rehab, they've put the stuffing back in me again, sort of. I use a cane now. Probably always will. My arm hurts sometimes for no apparent reason. At least I gained back some of the weight I lost. What a dope. Retirement wasn't supposed to be this way.

Union official — Perth-Amboy, N.J.

Points to ponder

- Most accidents can be prevented by not taking unnecessary risks.
- Before starting a project, ask yourself, what could go wrong and what's the safest way to do it.
- Don't be superman (or woman). Recognize your limitations.

What you can do

Learn the warning signals of diabetes. These can develop slowly and include excessive thirst, frequent urination, unexplained weight loss, blurred vision, recurring bladder, vaginal yeast and skin infections, slow healing sores, irritability, and tingling or loss of feeling in your hands or feet.

Eating a balanced diet, maintaining a healthy weight and staying active can help you prevent the onset of type 2 diabetes and help you manage the disease if you have it. To keep blood sugar within safe limits, monitor your blood sugar and take any medications your doctor prescribes. (See "Exercise," page 43, and "Nutrition," page 47.)

Your digestive system

Most of the changes that take place in your digestive system are so subtle that you may not notice them. Swallowing and the motions that automatically move digested food through the intestines slow down. The amount of surface area within your intestines diminishes slightly. The flow of secretions from your stomach, liver, pancreas and small intestine may decrease. These changes generally do not disrupt the digestive process.

Indigestion and heartburn. Indigestion is a nonspecific term used to describe discomfort in your abdomen, nausea and a bloated or full feeling after eating. A common form of indigestion is heartburn (gastroesophageal reflux disease, or GERD). Heartburn occurs when stomach acids back up into your food pipe (esophagus). A sour taste and the sensation of food coming back into your mouth may accompany a burning sensation behind your breastbone. Being overweight, smoking, overeating, and some medications, foods and beverages can all play a role in heartburn.

Excessive gas. The large intestine produces most intestinal gas. All people pass gas (flatulence), but some people produce an excessive amount of gas that bothers them throughout the day. Some older adults experience trouble digesting dairy products, a condition called lactose intolerance.

Constipation. This common problem is often misunderstood and improperly treated. Constipation is the passage of hard stools less than three times a week. In addition, passing stools may be difficult and painful. Many factors, including poor diet or diet changes, dehydration, medications, inactivity or illness can lead to constipation. Sometimes constipation is a symptom of an underlying disease, such as colon cancer or thyroid disorders.

What you can do

To prevent heartburn, slim down if you're overweight. Eat small, frequent meals, and stop eating 2 to 3 hours before you lie down or go to bed. Elevating the head of your bed by 4 to 6 inches may help.

Avoid heartburn-inducing food and drinks, including fatty foods, alcohol, caffeinated or carbonated beverages, decaffeinated coffee, peppermint, spearmint, garlic, onion, cinnamon, chocolate, citrus fruits and juices, and tomato products. Don't use nicotine.

Over-the-counter (OTC) antacids can help, but avoid using them for prolonged periods because they can cause diarrhea or constipation. When you take them before eating, acid-blocking medicines such as Pepcid, Tagamet and Zantac also may help. These are available in OTC and prescription strengths.

For more severe cases of reflux, two newer procedures are available to help tighten the valve that keeps stomach acids where they belong. (See "Nonsurgical procedures for heartburn relief," page 26.)

To reduce excessive flatulence, identify the foods that affect you the most. If dairy products bother you, try taking lactase tablets or drops (Lactaid or Dairy Ease) before eating these foods. Occasional use of OTC antigas products containing simethicone (Mylanta, Riopan Plus, Mylicon) or activated charcoal pills can help.

To lessen your chances of constipation, eat plenty of high-fiber foods, including fresh fruits, vegetables and whole-grain cereals and breads. Drink 8 to 10 glasses of water or other nonalcoholic liquids daily. Increase your physical activity. When you feel the urge to go to the bathroom, don't delay. Avoid commercial laxatives. Over time they can aggravate your constipation. Take fiber supplements such as Metamucil, Konsyl or Citrucel.

Colorectal cancer. Colorectal (ko-lo-REK-tul) cancer is the second leading cause of cancer deaths in the United States. Approximately 90 percent of people who develop this cancer are over age

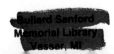

Nonsurgical procedures for heartburn relief

When lifestyle changes and medications don't provide acceptable relief for heartburn, newer nonsurgical procedures called endoscopic suturing and the Stretta system can help keep stomach acids from backing up into your food pipe.

During endoscopic suturing, a physician inserts an endoscope (a long tube) into your mouth and down your throat to reach the weakened band of muscles in your esophagus. A special tool allows the physician to place stitches in two different locations in the esophagus. Once inserted and tied, these stitches form barriers to block the passage of stomach acids into the esophagus.

The Stretta system uses controlled radio frequency energy to heat and melt tissues within the weakened valve at the junction of the stomach and the esophagus. It appears to work by creating scar tissue that helps tighten this valve.

Both of these procedures take an hour or less to perform and can generally be done without an overnight stay in the hospital. Their long-term effects are unknown.

50. Most colon cancers seem to develop from certain types of polyps, growths in the large intestines. Although polyps are relatively common, many are noncancerous (benign).

What you can do

Colon cancer usually grows very slowly. It may be present in your body for many years without producing recognizable symptoms. But early detection and treatment can save lives. That's why the American Cancer Society recommends colorectal screenings starting at age 50. If you have a family history of colon cancer or polyps, your doctor may recommend screenings beginning at an earlier age.

Your ears

Hearing loss. Although some people retain perfect hearing throughout their lives, most lose some hearing sensitivity gradually,

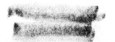

starting in their 20s. One-third of U.S. adults over age 65, nearly 10 million people, are hearing impaired. Age-related hearing loss first affects your ability to hear higher frequencies and by age 65 generally affects the lower frequencies also. Some people find it difficult to follow conversations in a crowded room or restaurant.

Changes that occur within the inner ear or in nerves attached to it, excess wax, and injuries caused by exposure to noise and various diseases can all impair your hearing. If hearing loss becomes significant, it can interfere with your safety as well as your social life.

What you can do

If you or a family member suspects that you have serious hearing loss, see a physician. Hearing loss can sometimes be restored with medical treatment or surgery, especially if the problem is in the outer ear or middle ear.

Hearing aids can't help everyone with hearing loss, but they can improve hearing for many people. These devices work by gathering in the sounds around you and making them louder. The problem is, they amplify all frequencies of sound, including unwanted noise. Newer digital hearing aids may reduce irritating background noise and provide the capability to fine-tune sound. However, no hearing aid can eliminate all background noise. Disposable hearing aids, which offer easier maintenance, also are available.

Here are some steps to follow if you're thinking of buying a hearing aid: Get a checkup and hearing examination to rule out correctable causes of hearing loss. Buy your hearing aid from a reputable dispenser and beware of misleading claims. Be cautious of "free" consultations and dispensers who sell only one brand of hearing aid. Make sure the hearing aid comes with a 30- to 60-day trial period, no penalty if you return it and a 1- to 2-year warranty covering parts and labor.

Dizziness. The word *dizzy* describes a variety of sensations, including a spinning sensation and a feeling of being faint, lightheaded, weak or unsteady on your feet. Although most of the causes of dizziness are benign, falling during one of these spells can result in broken bones and head injuries.

You may feel faint when you sit upright or stand too quickly because your blood pressure sometimes drops rapidly. Or you may feel this way after a coughing spell, if you're dehydrated or if you have heart disease or circulation problems. Anxiety disorders, medications and rapid breathing (hyperventilation) also can make you feel lightheaded.

A spinning sensation, called vertigo, usually results from a problem with the nerves and structures of your inner ear that sense position, movement and changes in your head position. In addition, viruses, alcohol and caffeine are sometimes to blame.

A loss of balance or a feeling of unsteadiness when you're walking has a variety of causes. Inner ear abnormalities, failing vision, nerve damage, arthritis, muscle weakness, general deconditioning and medications (especially seizure drugs, sedatives and tranquilizers) can all contribute to this problem.

What you can do

If you feel faint, sit down, lean forward and put your head between your knees or lie down and elevate your legs slightly. Changing positions slowly when you stand or sit upright can help prevent a rapid blood pressure drop. Drink plenty of liquids to avoid dehydration and promote good circulation. If you plan to be active in heat and humidity, dress to avoid overheating. Take breaks during the activity. Don't drive or use the stairs during a dizzy spell. Avoid smoking and alcohol.

If dizziness is a chronic problem, talk to your doctor. Most things that cause dizziness are not serious, but your doctor may want to review your medications and perform tests to pinpoint the cause.

Your eyes

Because good vision is a critical part of maintaining your independence, it's important to take care of your eyes. Like the rest of your body, your eyes change over time. They become less elastic and often become less able to focus on nearby objects. If you do not need glasses at least some of the time after age 65, you are the exception.

And vision loss increases with advancing age. More than one-quarter of people older than 85 report significant visual impairment.

Cataracts. Cataracts occur when the lenses in your eyes become cloudy or distorted. About half of Americans ages 65 to 75 have them to varying degrees. Cataracts sometimes cause blurred vision or double vision and typically create problems in night driving.

Glaucoma. Glaucoma is the buildup of fluid within the eyeball to an abnormally high pressure. This condition narrows your field of vision and can lead to blindness if not diagnosed and treated appropriately. Most people with this disease have no symptoms, but some will have pain or redness of the eyes and see colorful halos around lights. About 3 percent of people over 65 have glaucoma.

Macular degeneration. Macular degeneration is the leading cause of legal blindness among Americans older than age 65. This disease causes you to lose your central vision but maintain side (peripheral) vision. Its symptoms include hazy, gray vision and a central blind spot.

What you can do

Even if you don't have vision problems, as you age you'll need more light to see. Try using a flexible light, such as a gooseneck lamp, to direct light onto your reading or work. A variety of bifocal, trifocal and high-power eyeglasses are available to help you see more clearly. Magnification devices come in many styles, including hand-held, free-standing or attached to a chain that you can wear around your neck.

Large-print reading materials and devices, including locks, phones, playing cards and books, are available. Contact the American Foundation for the Blind, 11 Penn Plaza, Suite 300, New York, NY 10001; phone 212-502-7600 (*www.afb.org*).

The key to living with cataracts is knowing when it's time not to live with them anymore. Usually, this happens when your lifestyle becomes cramped because of your vision. If your cataracts have progressed to the point where you can't pass the vision test to renew your driver's license, it may be time to consider surgery. Fortunately, advanced surgical methods make cataract surgery one of the most successful procedures done today.

Routine eye exams and early detection are your best defense against glaucoma and macular degeneration. Early treatment, including surgery and medication, can help prevent significant visual loss from glaucoma.

No treatments can reverse damage already done by macular degeneration. Eating a balanced diet that contains plenty of green leafy vegetables, wearing sunglasses that block out harmful ultraviolet light and not smoking may decrease your risk of this disease. You can check yourself for signs and symptoms of macular degeneration by using an Amsler's grid (see below).

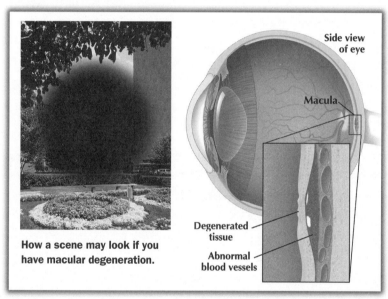

How a scene may look if you have macular degeneration.

Side view of eye

Macula

Degenerated tissue

Abnormal blood vessels

Macular degeneration is the deterioration of the macula, the small, central part of your retina. Sometimes it's caused by the growth of abnormal blood vessels under the macula.

An Amsler's grid is one test used for early detection of macular degeneration. To use the grid, hold it 12 to 15 inches away from your eyes in good light. Cover one eye (keep your reading glasses on). Look directly at the center dot. Note whether all lines of the grid are straight or if any areas are wavy, blurred or dark. Repeat with your other eye. If any area looks wavy, blurred or dark, contact your ophthalmologist.

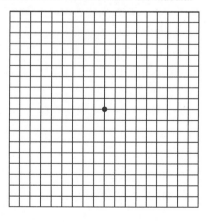

Your hair

Your hair changes with age, but individual variations are great. On average, half of us are about 50 percent gray by age 50. Graying usually begins at the temples and slowly works its way up the scalp. This gray hair is often different in texture. Underarm hair and pubic hair may not turn gray.

Some thinning of hair also typically occurs in both women and men. Men are more likely than women to have hair loss and baldness as they age. About 60 percent of men by age 50 experience hair loss or thinning. Male pattern baldness typically involves a receding hairline and hair loss on top of your head. Age, changing hormones and heredity cause some people to lose more hair than others.

A smaller number of women experience female pattern baldness as they age. Most women rarely develop bald patches. Your part may appear to widen, or your hair may look and feel thinner. Hormone alterations that occur after menopause sometimes cause facial hairs to coarsen and grow.

What you can do

If hair loss bothers you, several treatment options are available. Medications can stimulate growth of hair. Hair follicles can be surgically transplanted from other parts of your head. Toupees and weaves are other options. If facial hair is a problem, you can bleach it or remove it by plucking, waxing, electrolysis or with hair remover. Removal does not stimulate further growth.

Your heart and blood vessels

Even in the absence of any disease process, your heart and blood vessels change with age. Your heart muscle becomes less elastic and a less efficient pump, working harder to do the same job. Your heart may shrink and weigh slightly less than when you were young. There also may be some loss of the pacemaker cells that control your heart's activities.

Such changes in your cardiovascular system occur gradually rather than overnight. Despite these changes, your heart is strong enough to meet the normal needs of your body. It does, however, have less reserve capacity for overcoming injury or handling the sudden demands placed on it by stress or illness.

Coronary artery disease. Your blood vessels also become less elastic with age. Accumulations of deposits in the walls of your arteries, a condition called coronary artery disease (atherosclerosis), may make the passageway through your vessels narrow. Poor diet, genetics, inactivity, high blood pressure and smoking can accelerate this process.

Angina and heart attack. Narrowed arteries deprive the heart of oxygen and can result in pain called angina (an-JI-nuh). This can include pain or pressure in your chest and pain in your neck, jaw or arm. If the oxygen supply to your heart is restricted for more than 2 to 3 hours, blood-starved heart muscle tissue may actually die. This event is called myocardial infarction (MI) — a heart attack. (See "Heart attack symptoms," page 35.)

Congestive heart failure. Some people may not be aware that they have a heart problem until they develop symptoms of congestive heart failure — extreme fatigue with exertion and shortness of breath, especially when lying down. Congestive heart failure occurs when your heart is chronically weakened and can't pump enough blood to meet your body's demands. It often accompanies advanced stages of coronary artery disease.

High blood pressure. When you experience both loss of elasticity in your blood vessels and coronary artery disease, your heart must work harder to pump blood through a more resistant network of vessels. This effect can cause high blood pressure (hypertension), which makes your heart work even harder. Prolonged high blood pressure can damage your blood vessels, kidneys, heart or brain and cause death. Unfortunately, this condition rarely has any signs or symptoms.

What you can do

Heart disease and high blood pressure don't have to be deadly. You can take measures to prevent and manage these conditions.

Learn your risk factors. High blood cholesterol, diabetes, smoking, obesity, physical inactivity and family history can all put you at increased risk of heart disease and high blood pressure. By age 65 a woman's risk is almost equal to a man's. And blacks have a higher risk than whites, Hispanics or Asian Americans.

Exercise. Regular aerobic exercise, such as vigorous cycling, swimming, walking or jogging, may reduce LDL (low-density lipoprotein or "bad") cholesterol and triglycerides (fat), while increasing HDL (high-density lipoprotein or "good") cholesterol. It can also help increase your heart's capacity to pump and help keep your blood pressure in check. It reduces the risk of developing atherosclerosis. (See "Exercise," page 43.)

Stop smoking. Smoking raises your blood pressure and increases your risk of heart disease by at least two times.

Maintain a healthy weight. Losing excess weight helps reduce your risk of heart attack and high blood pressure.

Limit salt in your diet. Sodium in salt and salty foods causes your body to retain fluid and may increase your blood pressure. Try to limit sodium to no more than 2,400 milligrams a day, which is about a teaspoon of table salt.

Eat healthfully. Eating healthfully means reducing your intake of fat and cholesterol and eating more fruits and vegetables. Eat foods rich in folic acid, such as green leafy vegetables, citrus fruits, dried legumes, peanuts and cereal grains.

Limit alcohol. Regular consumption of small amounts of alcohol has been shown to lower the risk of heart attack. Experts recommend no more than one drink a day for women and one to two drinks a day for men.

Take medications. A variety of medications also may help prevent and control heart disease and high blood pressure. Simply taking one aspirin a day has been shown to reduce risk of a heart attack, but talk to your doctor about whether this is appropriate for you. If medications alone aren't sufficient to control coronary artery disease, your doctor may suggest surgical revascularization procedures, such as bypass surgery or angioplasty, to increase blood supply to your heart.

Your kidneys, bladder and urinary tract

Your kidneys. Each day your kidneys work to remove excess fluid and waste from your blood. They also produce important hormones and regulate the level of certain chemicals in your body.

Kidney function declines with age. At about age 40, you begin to lose some of the important filters within the kidneys, called nephrons (NEF-rons). This gradual decline in performance can be a problem if you're taking medications or if you have a chronic illness, such as high blood pressure or diabetes.

A severe decline or stop in function, called kidney failure, is becoming more common because people are living longer with chronic illnesses that can harm their kidneys. Once the damage is done, it's irreversible.

What you can do

To preserve kidney function, it's important to detect and treat as early as possible the conditions that can damage your kidneys. You can take several steps to slow and even stop the damage. Controlling high blood pressure and, if you have diabetes, blood sugar levels is necessary to protect your kidneys' health. Eating a low-salt, low-fat diet and taking in enough fluids also can help. Talk to your doctor about the safe use of over-the-counter (OTC) pain relievers. If you are at risk of or are already experiencing kidney failure, don't take large amounts of OTC pain relievers over a long period of time. Be sure to talk to your doctor about what other drugs and herbal supplements might be harmful to your kidneys.

Incontinence. A variety of factors can lead to incontinence. Excess weight, frequent constipation, a chronic cough and altered muscle activity within and around your bladder can all play a role. In men incontinence can stem from noncancerous enlargement of the prostate gland, prostate cancer and prostate surgery.

Following menopause, many women experience what's called stress incontinence as the muscles around the opening of the bladder (the sphincter muscles) lose strength. As estrogen levels decline, the tissues lining the tube through which urine passes (the urethra) become thinner. Pelvic muscles become weaker, reducing bladder support.

Other common causes of incontinence include urinary-related infections and diseases such as diabetes, stroke and Parkinson's disease, which can damage nerves that control your bladder.

Heart attack symptoms

The American Heart Association lists the following warning signs of heart attack. Be aware that you may not have them all, and symptoms may come and go. Seek medical treatment if you note any of these symptoms.

- Uncomfortable pressure, fullness, heaviness or squeezing pain in the center of your chest, lasting more than a few minutes
- Pain spreading to your shoulders, jaw, neck or arms
- Shortness of breath, lightheadedness, fainting, sweating or nausea.

Don't waste precious minutes because you fear your symptoms are a false alarm. Dial 911 or the emergency number in your area and ask for emergency transport. While you're waiting for emergency help to arrive, sit or lie down, breathe slowly and deeply, and chew an aspirin, unless you are allergic to it. Aspirin thins your blood and has been shown to significantly decrease death rates related to heart attacks.

Incontinence can also be caused by some medications for insomnia, depression, high blood pressure and heart disease.

What you can do

Lifestyle modifications can often help curb incontinence. You may be able to prevent accidents by using a fixed bathroom schedule rather than waiting for the need to go. Try limiting or avoiding alcohol and caffeine, which cause you to urinate more, and spicy or acidic foods, which can irritate your bladder. And crossing your legs when you feel a sneeze or a cough coming can sometimes help.

Pelvic floor exercises (Kegels) often help relieve mild to moderate stress incontinence in both women and men. To perform Kegels, imagine that you're trying to stop passing urine. Squeeze the muscles you would use and hold for a count of three. Relax for three counts, then repeat. Try to do this for about 5 minutes, three times a day.

If lifestyle changes aren't effective, medications, biofeedback and other treatments can help relieve incontinence. Hormone replacement therapy (HRT) may help incontinence resulting from menopausal changes. Sometimes surgery is necessary to improve the position of your bladder, add bulk to tissues or add support to weakened pelvic muscles.

Prostate disease. Found only in men, the prostate gland surrounds the bottom portion (neck) of the bladder. By the time men reach their senior years, a large number of them experience some type of prostate problem. Symptoms may range from minor and mildly annoying to serious and painful.

Noncancerous prostate enlargement. After age 45 or so, the prostate often begins to enlarge. This growth is called benign prostatic hyperplasia (pros-TAT-ik hy-pur-PLAY-zhuh), or BPH. As the gland enlarges, prostate tissue presses on the urethra and produces urinary problems. Many men first experience symptoms between ages 55 and 60. Others don't have symptoms until their 70s or 80s.

What you can do

Simple lifestyle changes can often help control symptoms of BPH and prevent your condition from worsening.

Limit beverages. Stop drinking liquids after 7 p.m. to reduce your need to use the bathroom at night.

Empty your bladder completely. Try to urinate all that you can each time you use the bathroom.

Limit alcohol. Limit your alcohol consumption because it increases urine production and may cause congestion in the prostate gland.

Be careful with over-the-counter decongestants. OTC decongestants can cause the muscle that controls urine flow to tighten, making urination more difficult.

Keep active. Inactivity causes you to retain urine.

Stay warm. Cold weather can lead to urinary urgency.

If your symptoms progress, your doctor may suggest medications or surgical correction.

Prostate cancer. As you age your risk of prostate cancer increases. It's estimated that by age 50, up to one in four men have some cancerous cells in the prostate gland. By age 80, the ratio increases to one in two.

Prostate cancer is the second leading cause of cancer deaths in American men — not because it's so deadly, but because it's so common. Unlike other cancers, you're more likely to die with prostate cancer than of it. On average, an American man has about a 30 percent risk of having prostate cancer, but only about a 3 percent risk of dying of the disease.

Unfortunately, prostate cancer produces few, if any, symptoms in its early stages. That's why it's important to have regular prostate checkups to catch the disease early.

Your lungs and respiratory system

To understand the effect of aging on your lungs, let's trace the path traveled by each breath you take. When you inhale, air enters your mouth and nose and travels through the back of your throat, through your voice box and down your windpipe (trachea). The trachea branches into two main air passageways, which branch into progressively smaller passageways and tubes called bronchioles. The smallest bronchioles end in tiny closed air sacs. Tiny blood vessels called pulmonary capillaries carry your blood to these air sacs, where they release carbon dioxide and absorb oxygen.

Healthy adult lungs contain approximately 300 million of these air sacs (alveoli). As you age, the number of these air sacs decreases. If you're healthy, you probably won't notice this gradual change, especially if you lead an active life.

Chronic breathing problems. Some older adults gradually develop chronic breathing difficulties, including chronic bronchitis and emphysema. In chronic bronchitis, the lining of your bronchial tubes becomes chronically inflamed. Emphysema, also called chronic obstructive pulmonary disease (COPD), occurs when the smaller bronchial passages become damaged. Smoking over a long period is the main cause of both of these problems. In some cases long-term exposure to chemical fumes, dusts or other irritants also can play a role.

A price to pay

I must confess I let my health slide. I say confess because I'm a physician and should know better. I entered residency sleek as a greyhound at 155 pounds. By age 50, I weighed 205. I seldom exercised, smoked a half a pack of cigarettes a day and got winded when I walked a couple flights of stairs. I would like to sound noble by suggesting I was too busy taking care of other people to take care of myself. That's true, but the heart of the matter is I felt invincible and was caught up in my own success. The price I paid for that success was physical and mental exhaustion. Burnout: I had it big-time.

I was a prominent orthopedic surgeon who attracted a high-profile global clientele. It felt good to be invited to speak at conferences where more than once I was introduced as one of the most technically gifted surgeons in America. I rather enjoyed seeing my name listed as principle investigator on numerous peer-reviewed papers. They sent me the most difficult cases, as well as prominent, affluent people for whom a bad outcome could cost the institution bad publicity. I was good, but also arrogant. And so it went for twenty years.

Perhaps I'm scapegoating, but my career began to crumble the day I woke up and managed care was staring me in the face. Reimbursement restrictions meant we physicians had to perform more procedures to make up for the loss of revenue. Our travel and conference budgets were significantly decreased. To be given performance quotas was humiliating and stressful for us all.

Respiratory infections. Older adults are also more vulnerable to respiratory infections such as influenza (flu), pneumonia and tuberculosis (TB). Although these infections are not always serious, each year flu and pneumonia cause about 45,000 deaths in the United States. The majority of the people who die are older than age 65. People with chronic heart or lung

Younger colleagues seemed to adapt. Many of the old guard did as well. I simply found myself physically and psychologically exhausted by the whole ordeal. I battled with administration in an effort to get some of my former autonomy back. But they spoke to me in a foreign language about productivity, scheduling gaps and "meeting departmental expectations." The final blow came when, barely having the energy to make it through the day, I was told I was not doing my share.

In an attempt to survive the grind long enough to exit with dignity, I requested a 4-day workweek, with salary adjusted accordingly. They agreed, reluctantly, but it was a miscalculation on my part. They crammed 5 days of patients into 4 days, so I was earning less for the privilege of being more exhausted than when I was working 5 days a week. Instead of my operating schedule starting at 8:30, I was to be gowned and scrubbed for my first patient by 7. I often ponder whether I would've gotten along better with the changes had my stamina been up to snuff. I'll never know. The only certainty is that it was time for me to hang up my white coat.

Surgeon — San Diego, Calif

Points to ponder

- Staying fit is job No. 1. Good health is the cornerstone to successful aging.

- Our capacity for work and leisure enjoyment is directly related to our physical, psychological and spiritual health.

disorders are at increased risk.

TB was common in the United States before 1940. If you were exposed to the disease then, you can harbor inactive or dormant TB bacteria that reactivate later in life when your resistance is weakened.

What you can do

To protect your lungs and respiratory system, stop smoking and eliminate smoke from your environment. If you're 65 or older, get pneumonia and influenza vaccinations. Flu vaccines need to be repeated each year. Getting regular exercise and maintaining a healthy weight can reduce the strain on your lungs and help keep them fit.

Your skin

Your skin shows its age by losing some of its elasticity. This causes drooping. You can keep the underlying muscles firm and taut, but in some places, such as your face, your skin will sag and wrinkle anyway. Your skin also becomes a little thinner, so that veins or discolorations beneath the surface show through more clearly than they used to. You begin to lose your youthful color and glow. Decreased production of natural oils makes your skin drier, and you probably perspire less.

If you are white, age spots, also known as liver spots, probably will appear. These small, flat patches look like freckles. Although age spots are harmless, see your physician if you observe changes in an existing growth on your skin or a sore that doesn't heal, just to rule out skin cancer.

Tiny blood vessels just below the surface of the skin may become fragile, break and bleed. This causes superficial bruising, a condition called senile purpura. It occurs mainly on the forearms.

The loss of natural skin oils can cause intense itching on your back, lower legs, hands or elsewhere. This condition is called asteatosis, and it produces scaly skin that sometimes cracks deeply.

How fast your skin ages depends on many factors. The most significant of these is how much unprotected exposure to the sun you have had over the years. The more sun, the more damage you can expect. Smoking also is an enemy to your skin. It slows your skin's ability to heal and causes paleness, yellowing and deep wrinkles around your lips.

Skin cancer. At this stage in your life, you can't undo years of exposure to the sun. But you can learn how to recognize the early signs of skin cancer so that treatment can begin early.

Melanoma is the deadliest form of skin cancer. The ABCD rule can help you tell a normal mole from one that could be melanoma:

- **A** stands for asymmetrical shape. Look for irregular shapes. Symmetrical round or oval growths are usually noncancerous.

- **B** is for border irregularity. Irregular, notched, scalloped or poorly defined borders need a closer look.

- **C** is for color. Look for growths that have many colors or an uneven distribution of color.

- **D** is for diameter. Have your doctor examine any growth larger in diameter than a pencil eraser, about a quarter inch.

Be sure to keep an eye on moles located around your nails or genitals, and those that have been present since birth. In addition, rapid-growing, bleeding and nonhealing sores could be symptoms of skin cancer.

What you can do

Good skin care throughout life is your best weapon against wrinkles, dryness and skin cancer. Stay out of the sun or apply sunscreen to protect your skin from the ultraviolet rays of sunlight. Don't smoke. Nicotine in cigarette smoke constricts the blood vessels that nourish your skin. Like other organs, your skin also benefits from a good blood supply provided by a healthy diet and regular exercise.

To relieve dryness and itching, take fewer baths or showers, avoid antibacterial soaps, don't wear wool clothes, increase the humidity in your home during winter and apply oils to your skin. Moisturizers applied after bathing can't prevent wrinkles, but they can temporarily mask tiny lines and creases that detract from the appearance of your skin. Remember that pricey products or scientific-sounding ingredients are no guarantee of greater effectiveness.

Despite all the hype about antioxidant creams and topical vitamins, there's little evidence that they improve your skin. What does help is Retin-A, a prescription cream containing retinoic acid, a synthetic derivative of vitamin A. It's not a miracle drug, but it has been shown to decrease fine wrinkling, roughness and pigment changes in mildly to moderately affected skin.

Your teeth and gums

How your teeth and gums respond to age depends on how well you've cared for them over the years. But even if you're meticulous about brushing and flossing, you may notice that your mouth feels drier and your gums have receded (pulled back). Your teeth may darken slightly and become more brittle and easier to break.

With less saliva to wash away bacteria, your teeth and gums become slightly more vulnerable to decay and infection. Smoking, illness and certain medications can aggravate these problems. Mild gum disease makes your gums red, puffy and sore. Left untreated, gum disease can progress until your teeth loosen and fall out.

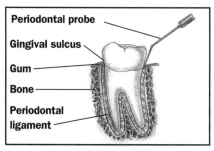

Your dentist uses a periodontal probe to measure the depth of your sulcus.

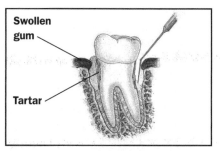

An accumulation of tartar can lead to gingivitis, characterized by swollen gums.

Denture sores are usually due to improper fit. If you've worn your dentures for a while and begin developing sores, this irritation may indicate a change in the denture or in the alignment of your mouth. If your weight changes, your dentures may need to be refitted. Sores can also develop if food becomes trapped beneath the dentures. In rare cases recurrent mouth sores can signal a health problem.

What you can do

Brush at least twice daily and floss daily. Be sure to clean both the outer and inner surfaces of your teeth and gums. If you have difficulty performing these tasks, brushing with an electric toothbrush and using floss aids can help.

If you're having problems with denture sores, see your dentist to have your dentures adjusted. To avoid sores caused by trapped food, brush after every meal, take out your dentures at night and brush your gums, tongue and palate. Avoid using an over-the-counter ointment to numb denture-sore pain. In addition to daily oral care, visit your dentist at least annually for a routine cleaning and dental checkup.

Preserving your lifestyle

In this section, we'll discuss some strategies that can help you prevent, minimize or cope with the age-related changes presented earlier in this chapter.

Exercise

There was a time when older adults were expected to sit and watch life from the sidelines. But today many are trading their rockers and recliners for athletic shoes. The reason? Physical fitness pays. Regular exercise can help prevent coronary artery disease, high blood pressure, stroke, diabetes, depression, falls and some cancers. And fitness reduces the lifestyle-limiting effects of osteoporosis and arthritis.

Research shows that exercise can slow the loss of bone and increase the size and strength of your muscles, including your heart. Exercise helps prevent loss of aerobic capacity, the ability of your heart, lungs and blood vessels to deliver adequate oxygen to your muscles during physical activity. If you are inactive your aerobic capacity will decrease by half or more by the time you reach 80. In contrast, one study showed that active older adults lost only a small percentage of their aerobic capacity by age 70.

Being physically fit can keep you stronger and give you better balance, flexibility and coordination. All of these benefits can help you remain more independent as you age. The bottom line — fitness can improve the quality of your life.

Getting started. You can begin exercising at any age, even if you've never exercised before. But before you do anything more vigorous than walking, see your doctor. This is especially important if you've been inactive for some time, if you have a family history of heart disease, if you have heart or lung disease, or if you are unsure about your health. Also check with your doctor if you have high blood pressure, diabetes, arthritis or asthma, or if you smoke. Ask your doctor about how your medications may affect your exercise plan.

Planning your program. The "no pain, no gain" attitude toward exercise is a thing of the past. Forget it. Whether you exercise at home, in a pool or at a club, the best fitness programs start slowly and gradually increase in intensity. Experts now recommend a combination of stretching (flexibility) exercises, aerobic (endurance) exercise and strength training (weight training). Your workout should also include time to warm up and cool down. Listen to your body during and after workouts for signs that you may have a health problem as a result of overexertion. (See "Danger signs during exercise," page 47.)

Stretching exercises. Flexibility exercises can help you counteract joint and muscle stiffness, maintain your joint range of motion and prevent injury. These exercises also make everyday activities like tying shoes easier. Stretching doesn't require special equipment or a lot of time. Warm up first with a low-intensity exercise like walking and gently pumping your arms. Do stretching exercises for 5 to 10 minutes before and, more importantly, after each aerobic exercise session. Don't bounce, and remember that prolonged (20- to 30-second) stretching is most effective.

Aerobic exercise. Moderate-intensity exercise such as hiking, stair climbing, aerobic dancing, jogging, bicycling, rowing and swimming help improve your aerobic capacity. But if you're just getting started, try lower intensity activities like walking or cycling.

Weight-bearing activities, which include any activity you do on your feet with your bones supporting your weight, help strengthen your bones. Exercises that involve repeated impact have added benefit. These include walking, dancing, stair climbing, skipping rope, skiing and racket sports.

Vary your activities so that you exercise both your upper and lower body. The frequency and duration of activity are more important than the intensity. Aim for 20 to 40 minutes of moderate exercise, 5 or more days a week.

Recommended stretches

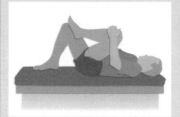

LOWER BACK STRETCH. Lie on a firm surface, such as the floor or a table, with your hips and knees bent and feet flat on the surface. Pull your left knee toward your left shoulder with both hands (if you have knee problems, pull from the back of your thigh). Hold for 30 seconds. Relax. Repeat with other leg.

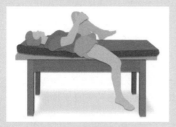

UPPER THIGH STRETCH. Lie on a table or bed with one leg and hip as near the edge as possible and your lower leg hanging relaxed over the edge. Pull your other thigh and knee firmly toward your chest until your lower back flattens against the table. Hold for 30 seconds. Relax. Repeat with other leg.

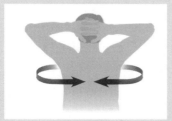

CHEST STRETCH. Clasp your hands behind your head. Pull elbows firmly back while inhaling deeply. Hold for 30 seconds (keep breathing). Relax.

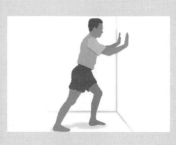

CALF STRETCH. Stand arm's-length from wall. Lean into wall. Place one leg forward with knee bent. Keep other leg back with knee straight and heel down. Keeping back straight, move hips toward wall until you feel a stretch. Hold 30 seconds. Relax. Repeat with other leg.

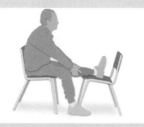

HAMSTRING STRETCH. Sit in a chair with one leg on another chair. Keep back straight. Slowly bend pelvis forward at the hip until you feel a stretch in the back of your thigh. Hold 30 seconds. Relax. Repeat with other leg.

Recommended strength exercises

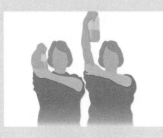

TRICEPS EXTENSION. Slowly lift a weight above your head as shown. Lower weight to starting position. Repeat 10 to 12 times. Relax. Repeat with your other arm. Increase weight and repetitions as your muscles become stronger.

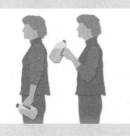

ARM CURL. Place your feet shoulder-width apart. Keep upper arm straight and flex your elbow until the weight is shoulder height. Hold, then lower weight slowly. Repeat 10 to 12 times, then exercise other arm. Increase weight and repetitions as your muscles become stronger.

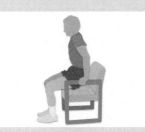

CHAIR SIT-UPS. Sit in a chair that has arms. Push your body up off the surface of the chair using your arms only. Hold 10 seconds. Relax and repeat.

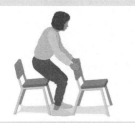

CHAIR SITS. Set up two chairs as shown. Hold onto the chair in front of you. Begin to sit in the chair behind you in a position you can hold for 10 seconds. As you build strength, try to hold a lower position that is almost, but not quite, seated. Hold 10 seconds. Relax and repeat.

Danger signs during exercise

Stop exercising and seek immediate medical care if you have any of these signs: tightness in your chest, severe shortness of breath, chest pain, pain in your arms or jaw (often on the left side), palpitations (a thumping feeling in your heart), dizziness, faintness or a feeling of being sick to your stomach.

Strength training. Doing the simplest of strength exercises a couple of times each week can help you build stronger muscles and bones and control your weight. You can use weight machines or free weights, such as dumbbells, weight cuffs and homemade weights. Start with weights that are light enough to enable you to do 8 to 15 repetitions. As you gain strength, gradually increase the weight and decrease the number of repetitions until you're doing 12 repetitions and the 12th is at maximum effort.

Cooling down. At the end of your aerobic exercise or strength-training session, cool down with low-intensity movement (like walking or marching in place) until your heart rate returns to normal. Then repeat your stretching exercises, holding each stretch for 30 to 45 seconds.

Nutrition

Numerous studies show that a healthful diet, when combined with exercise and regular mental activity, can help you live longer and better. But physical changes and other factors that sometimes accompany aging mean that you may have to alter your approach to nutrition. As your metabolism slows down with age, your calorie needs decrease. To help you make sound eating choices, here are some guiding principles:

Increase your fiber intake. A high-fiber diet can help prevent constipation and may decrease your risk of some colon problems, including colon cancer. In addition, it helps protect against diabetes, heart disease and high blood pressure. Mayo Clinic nutritionists suggest getting 25 to 30 grams of fiber a day from a variety of foods. Go for whole-grain foods, like high-fiber cereals or whole-wheat breads, and whole foods, such as a fresh apple instead of apple juice. Read labels to get the maximum amount of fiber. Substitute legumes, such as beans or lentils, for meat a couple of times a week.

Drink plenty of fluids. As you get older, your thirst mechanism declines. Inadequate fluid intake sets you up for problems that may include chronic constipation, low blood pressure, impaired kidney function and kidney stones. Aim for at least eight glasses a day of nonalcoholic liquids, preferably water.

Choose nutrient-dense foods. Get the most out of every calorie you consume by choosing foods that contain a lot of nutrients in relation to their calories. Richly colored fruits and vegetables offer lots of essential nutrients. Whole-grain breads, rice, cereals and pastas contain more fiber compared to enriched or refined products. They also contain more of some vitamins and minerals. Don't replace a balanced diet with liquid supplements. Use them to boost rather than replace a healthy diet.

Anti-aging remedies, vitamins and dietary supplements

It's not likely that one product, pill or potion could be a cure for all the ills age can bring. Despite tempting claims, no product has been proven to prevent or reverse aging.

Some remedies have potentially dangerous side effects. Even though they may not be labeled drugs, nonprescription remedies such as vitamins, herbs, dietary supplements and hormones can interact with the medications you may be taking. That's why it's essential to talk to your doctor before you take any home remedy or store-bought treatments.

Because they're exempt from federal safety evaluations that drugs undergo, vitamins and other dietary supplements sold without prescriptions are not guaranteed to be safe. The bottom line is buyer beware.

Sexuality

Like adults of all ages, you probably want to continue sharing your life with others in fulfilling relationships. And you may want to include sex in an intimate relationship with someone you love. The idea that your sex drive dissolves sometime after middle age is simply a myth. The reality is that today's older adults enjoy an active sex life that often is better than their sex life in early adulthood.

Changes in women. Desire is the most variable of your sexual responses. Your sex drive is largely determined by emotional and social factors. Surprisingly, your sexual desire is affected mainly by the hormone testosterone, produced in your adrenal glands, rather than estrogen. Even though women's estrogen levels decline following menopause, most women produce enough testosterone to preserve their interest in sex.

Estrogen deficiency after menopause can slow the swelling and lubrication of the vagina during arousal. This can make intercourse less comfortable or even painful. And women in their 60s and 70s have a greater incidence of painful uterine contractions during orgasm. Hysterectomy (removal of the uterus and cervix) does not usually affect sexual pleasure.

What you can do

Sexual arousal begins in your brain. Depending on your personal preference, candlelight, music, food, conversation, books and thoughts can help you create a mood for sexual intimacy.

Longer foreplay sometimes helps stimulate your natural lubrication. Try a water-based lubricant such as K-Y jelly (not Vaseline or other petroleum-based jellies) or talk to your doctor about estrogen cream or estrogen replacement therapy. Having intercourse regularly also helps you maintain vaginal lubrication and elasticity.

Changes in men. Physical changes in men's sexual response parallel those in women. The great majority of aging men produce enough testosterone to maintain their interest in sex. But you may need more physical and mental stimulation to get and maintain an erection. Your erections may be less firm and may not last as long. And aging increases the time between possible ejaculations. By the time you reach age 70, it could take as much as 48 hours.

What you can do

Accepting changes and talking with your partner about them is important. Using a position that makes it easy to insert the penis into the vagina can help. Condoms can reduce stimulation, so don't wear one unless necessary to prevent conception or disease transmission.

If you have problems maintaining an erection or reaching orgasm, talk to your physician, who can help you and your partner understand the normal changes of aging and how to adapt to them.

Sildenafil (Viagra), self-injection therapy, penile vacuum pumps and other medications can help some men produce and maintain an erection. Viagra enhances the response to sexual stimulation by helping improve blood flow to the penis. But this drug can be dangerous — even lethal — if mixed with several common medications, or if you have coronary artery disease. Don't take Viagra without thoroughly discussing your health with your doctor. And never order "Viagra" over the Internet. It may not be the same product.

Vacuum devices, vascular surgery and surgical implants are other alternatives to help produce an erection.

Changes due to illness or disability. Some medical problems can interfere with how you respond sexually to another person. Chronic pain or surgery and illness that cause fatigue can make sexual activities more challenging or painful.

Chest pain, shortness of breath or the fear of a recurring heart attack can affect your desire and ability. But if you were sexually active before your heart attack, you can probably resume this activity. Sudden death during sex is rare.

Coronary artery disease and diabetes can restrict blood flow to your genitals. This can interfere with erection in men and the swelling of vaginal tissues in women. Men who have had diabetes for many years may also have nerve damage that can lead to impotence.

Some commonly used medications can interfere with sexual function. Drugs that control high blood pressure can reduce desire and impair erection in men and lubrication in women. Alcohol, antihistamines, antidepressants and acid-blocking drugs can have side effects that affect sexual function.

What you can do

Talk to your physician about how your health condition or medications can affect your sexual abilities. Find out what measures you can take to lessen the impact. Keep communicating with your partner about what does and does not feel good, and make adjustments to help create pleasure and avoid pain. If intercourse is not possible, learn to find pleasure in touch and other intimate activities.

Sleep

Your need for sleep remains fairly constant throughout most of your life. If you need about 6 hours nightly now, chances are you'll need that amount, give or take a half-hour, 10 years from now. However, aging can cause you to sleep less soundly.

Between ages 50 and 60, sleep often becomes less restful. You spend less time in deep sleep (called delta sleep). You also get tired earlier in the evening and wake up earlier in the morning.

If you think you're sleeping less, remember to count afternoon naps. Many older people who rest during the day find that the combination of naps and nighttime sleep totals just about the same hours of rest they had when they were younger.

Insomnia does become more prevalent with age. Changes in your sleep patterns, activity level and health can disrupt your sleep schedule. Chronic pain, depression, anxiety and stress also can interfere with sleep. Men who develop noncancerous enlargement of the prostate have their sleep interrupted by the need to urinate more frequently. Medications, including some antidepressants, high blood pressure medicines and steroid medicines, also can be at fault. And a snoring bed partner may interfere with your ability to get a good night's sleep.

What you can do

Lack of sleep, or insomnia, isn't an inevitable part of aging. Sleep experts offer the following tips to help you get a better night's sleep.

Minimize your interruptions. Close your door or create a subtle background noise like a fan to drown out other noises. If you drink less before bed, you won't need to use the bathroom as often.

Limit your naps and time in bed. This can help you avoid shallow, unrestful sleep.

Exercise daily. Finish your workout at least 5 to 6 hours before bedtime.

Avoid or limit substances that can disrupt your sleep cycle. These include caffeine, alcohol and nicotine.

Wind down gradually. Decrease stimuli just before bedtime. Take a warm shower or bath. Read a book or watch television until you become drowsy.

Be careful about medications. Talk to your doctor before taking any sleeping pills, especially if you are taking other prescription medications. And ask whether your medications may contribute to insomnia.

Coping with snoring

Snoring can deprive you and your bed partner of a good night's sleep. More common in men than in women, chronic snoring can leave you feeling drowsy during the day.

Here are tips to reduce or eliminate snoring:

- Lose excess weight. Even a 10 percent loss may help relieve snoring caused by constriction or obstruction of your windpipe.
- Avoid alcohol and medications such as tranquilizers and sleeping pills.
- Sleep on your side or stomach rather than your back. This helps keep your tongue from blocking your airway during sleep.

Some chronic snorers have a disorder called sleep apnea. The most common form of sleep apnea is when the muscles in the walls of your throat relax while you sleep so that the walls collapse and temporarily obstruct the flow of air. If your bed partner notices a periodic cessation of breathing, see your doctor. This condition can contribute to high blood pressure and heart damage.

Chapter 3

Your mind

- **A slip in memory does not signal Alzheimer's disease.**
- **Depression can be treated effectively.**
- **Your mind is like muscle, use it or lose it.**

I t isn't fair, is it? Just when you're old enough to have acquired some wisdom, your mind starts to play tricks on you. You can't remember where you left your glasses or where you parked your car. You used to be able to do three things at once, but now you're hard-pressed to focus on one. Some days, your lack of concentration is so pronounced, you fear that you have Alzheimer's disease. What's going on, and is there anything you can do about it?

First of all, relax. Some memory slippage is normal as you age. Misplacing your car keys or forgetting a name on occasion, though frustrating, isn't necessarily serious. Second of all, a number of conditions, such as depression and high blood pressure, and some medications can affect memory. Often the memory loss they cause is reversible.

Here's another good reason to relax: Stress and anxiety can interfere with your memory and your concentration.

In this chapter, we'll review memory loss. We'll look at the difference between simple memory loss and a progressive form of memory loss called dementia. We'll tell you what you can do to keep your mind active and alert throughout your later years. We'll start by looking at depression, a frequent cause of memory woes.

Beyond blue

We all feel blue from time to time, and everyone experiences grief. But depression is different. It's a serious illness that can take a terrible toll on the people who experience it, and their families. It's normal to feel sad at times, especially following a difficult loss, such as the death of a loved one. But unlike the blues, depression doesn't let go very easily. It won't go away in a few days or even weeks. In fact, if major depression is left untreated, it is likely to hang on from 6 to 24 months. And after the symptoms abate, they usually recur.

Depression is a medical disorder with a biological basis. It affects your thoughts, moods, feelings, behavior and physical health. Scientists believe it may be linked to imbalances in brain chemicals called neurotransmitters, particularly the neurotransmitters serotonin, norepinephrine and dopamine. But they don't fully understand the role these chemicals play in depression.

Despite all that we know about depression being a medical disorder, for some people there's still a stigma attached to it as a mental illness. Being depressed is no more cause for embarrassment than having diabetes or the flu, yet many people who are depressed feel ashamed or weak. They think, and are often told by others, that they should be able to snap out of it or that their suffering is all in their head. Often shame and embarrassment keep them from seeking the help they need.

Depression is more common in women than in men, affecting about one in four women, possibly because of biological causes such as hormones. It's less common among married people, especially married men, and those in long-term, intimate relationships. Depression rates are higher among those who are divorced, those who live alone and those who have difficulty with alcohol.

Like memory loss, depression isn't a natural part of aging. It's not more common among older people, but because some of the symptoms often are mistaken for inevitable consequences of growing older, it's more likely to go unrecognized in older adults. That's a serious concern because untreated depression can lead to a downward spiral of disability, dependency and suicide.

Also, a number of aspects of aging may predispose older adults to depression. These include decreases in neurotransmitter and hormone levels, loss of friends, loss of stature in the community, loss of work connections, loss of loved ones, moving out of a beloved home or the onset of chronic illnesses, such as heart disease, stroke, arthritis and diabetes.

There's no single cause for depression. Experts think some people have a genetic vulnerability to it, meaning the condition tends to run in families. That combined with stressful life events, such as the death of a spouse, the loss of a job, financial troubles or physical illness, may trigger a neurotransmitter imbalance that results in depression.

Your personality may predispose you to depression. Personality traits such as low self-esteem and being overly dependent, self-critical, pessimistic and easily overwhelmed by stress may make you more vulnerable. This doesn't mean you're a weak person.

Exaggerated anxiety often accompanies depression. An anxiety disorder can take a number of different forms, including generalized anxiety disorder, panic disorder and obsessive-compulsive disorder. With an anxiety disorder, you may feel apprehension, nervousness and a nagging uneasiness about your future. In some people anxiety mimics a heart attack, with symptoms such as a rapid heartbeat, palpitations, sweating and dizziness. Other symptoms include headaches, insomnia and fatigue.

Like depression, anxiety disorders may run in families and be linked to an imbalance in neurotransmitters. If you're experiencing anxiety as part of your depression, then the symptoms may be relieved when the depression subsides. If you have an anxiety disorder without depression, some of the same medications used for depression still may be effective. Relaxation techniques also can help. The important thing is, if you have symptoms either of depression or anxiety, don't assume it's a normal part of aging or that you can't do anything about it. Talk to your doctor.

Alcohol, nicotine and drug abuse contribute to depression and anxiety disorders. Diet can play a part, too. Specifically, deficiencies in folate and vitamin B-12 can cause symptoms of depression.

Are you depressed?

How do you know whether you're depressed? Depression has two hallmarks. One is loss of interest in normal daily activities. The other is a depressed mood, including feelings of sadness, helplessness and hopelessness, that lasts more than 2 weeks. As mentioned previously, many people with depression feel anxious as well.

For a doctor to diagnose depression, other signs and symptoms also must be present most of the day, nearly every day, for at least 2 weeks. They include memory problems and the inability to concentrate, sleep disturbances, significant weight loss or gain, fatigue, thoughts of death, agitation and loss of interest in sex.

Other physical symptoms associated with depression include headaches, constipation, diarrhea, abdominal pain and general aches and pains. People who are depressed may appear tired and may talk softly and slowly, as though they can barely muster the energy to speak.

Drs. Javaid I. Sheikh and Jerome A. Yesavage developed the Geriatric Depression Scale, a short form of which follows. If you think you or a loved one may be depressed, this questionnaire can help you decide whether to seek medical help. Answer yes or no to the questions, or if you are concerned about your loved one's health, have him or her do so:

1. Are you basically satisfied with your life?
2. Have you dropped many of your activities and interests?
3. Do you feel your life is empty?
4. Do you often get bored?
5. Are you in good spirits most of the time?
6. Are you afraid something bad is going to happen to you?
7. Do you feel happy most of the time?
8. Do you often feel helpless?
9. Do you prefer to stay at home rather than going out and doing new things?
10. Do you feel that you have more problems with memory than most people?
11. Do you think it's wonderful to be alive now?
12. Do you feel pretty worthless the way you are now?
13. Do you feel full of energy?
14. Do you feel your situation is hopeless?
15. Do you think that most people are better off than you are?

If you answered yes to questions 1, 5, 7, 11 and 13, you probably aren't depressed. Answering yes to most or all of the other questions strongly suggests depression. Talk to your doctor about your symptoms. You don't need to suffer. The sooner you get help, the better.

The best news about depression is that it's treatable. Over the past 20 years, medications have been developed that can relieve symptoms in most people. These include selective serotonin reuptake inhibitors (SSRIs), such as fluoxetine (Prozac), paroxetine (Paxil), sertraline (Zoloft) and citalopram (Celexa). But these are just some of the numerous antidepressants available. Medication choice depends on your illness, symptoms and your personal or family history of depression.

As with all medications, there are some cautions, especially for older people. As you get older, drugs clear from your body more slowly, so you may require lower doses. Your doctor will need to monitor your dosage carefully. He or she also needs to know whether you're taking other medications because they may interact with antidepressants. Antidepressants that cause sedation can make you prone to falls or other accidents.

Some people can discontinue the medication after 12 months. Others, whose depression tends to recur, might have to stay on it for years. The longer you stay on it, the less likely the depression is to recur. Antidepressant medications are not addictive.

Psychotherapy (talk therapy) also can help people with mild to moderate depression. In fact, psychotherapy and medication combined are more effective than either treatment alone. Both psychotherapy and medication can take 4 to 8 weeks to take effect, so you have to have patience and try not to get more upset because you think the treatment isn't working. For severe depression, electroconvulsive therapy (ECT) is the most effective option.

Taking care of your health can affect depression. Recent studies have shown that regular physical activity helps ward off or relieve the symptoms of depression in older adults.

For more information, see our Web site at *www.MayoClinic.com* and search on the word *depression*.

Unnatural losses

Let's get to the bottom line. When it comes to memory loss, most people's greatest fear is dementia, particularly the dementia that accompanies Alzheimer's disease.

A progressive and incurable brain disorder, Alzheimer's disease causes memory loss, changes in behavior and personality, and a decline in cognitive abilities. Symptoms typically appear after age 60. The disease becomes so debilitating that many people end up bedridden and die of pneumonia or other illnesses or infections within a decade after diagnosis.

Alzheimer's disease is a devastating illness that affects 4 million Americans and costs society an estimated $50 billion a year. The number of people with the disease is expected to triple in the next 20 years. More women than men are affected, although no one knows why. Women live longer, and the risk of developing

Alzheimer's increases with age, but that doesn't fully explain it.

But here's the better news: Because the disease affects so many people and burdens society, a tremendous amount of research on it is being conducted. As a result the past decade has brought great leaps in understanding the disease. There's also encouraging progress in early diagnosis and treatment of symptoms, as well as hope for a vaccine. Pretty amazing when you realize that 25 years ago medical science knew almost nothing about Alzheimer's disease and considered dementia to be an inevitable consequence of aging.

The changes in your mind related to Alzheimer's occur slowly, with degeneration often taking a decade. Mild forgetfulness, similar to what most of us experience, leads to problems finding the right word. Again, that's a pretty common experience. But with Alzheimer's the losses keep coming. You might notice behavior changes such as apathy, withdrawal or agitation. You may frequently forget what day, week, month or year it is. Your ability to do math may decline. Your finances may be a mess, with unpaid bills or overdrawn accounts. Driving may become more difficult and risky. Your family may notice that you frequently repeat questions or forget things. Eventually, the disease robs you of the ability not only to recognize common objects, such as a pencil, but also to use them. As the disease progresses and the dementia becomes more pro-nounced, independent living becomes impossible. It's like the lights going out in the house, one by one. It's a long goodbye.

Of course, Alzheimer's isn't the only cause of dementia. Another common cause is small strokes or changes in the brain's blood sup-ply that may kill brain tissue. This is known as vascular dementia (multi-infarct dementia). Symptoms of this type of dementia may come on suddenly and improve or remain stable until another stroke occurs. The location of the strokes in the brain determines the seriousness of the symptoms.

A difficult diagnosis. One of the peculiarities of Alzheimer's disease is that it's impossible to pinpoint the diagnosis without an autopsy. That's why the disease is sometimes referred to as probable

Only human

I was so cocky back then. When you're young you think you're Teflon coated. There's nothing you can't handle. But as the years went by, I learned I was human just like everyone else. I'm very grateful to those who were there to help, and I'm grateful I had the guts to ask for their help.

At age 20, I signed on with the company right out of tech school. Mainframes were as hot back then as laptops, servers and personal digital assistants are now. I worked with a bunch of young, hungry Turks who knew their salt. We had the technical staff and marketing savvy to keep us at the top. I flew to Italy, Singapore and Tokyo like others commute across town. I'd stay awake for 2 days reviewing business plans and solving technical challenges. For me it was a badge of honor and in hindsight kind of a macho ego thing, too.

I guess I was moving so fast I didn't notice when the wheels started falling off. New competitors were more nimble. They chipped away at our market share. Demand for mainframes was slumping at the same time. I had to watch my buddies clean out their desk and walk out the door pink slip in hand. Still, I thought, not me, not after what I've given to this company. Of course I got the ax just like the rest. There I was, 54 years old and on the street, with obsolete technical skills nobody wanted and competing with youngsters half my age. I was counting on consulting work to keep me busy, but the phone never rang, and my e-mail box stayed empty. Out of sight, out of mind. Damaged goods. A running back with a knee injury.

My wife was working full time while I stayed home with the cat. Summers were OK. I could always find a golf partner or tootle around on the boat. It was that second winter I started drinking — a couple eye-openers in the morning, a few pick-me-ups in the afternoon. Seventy channels on cable and next thing I knew it was dark.

My father, who was in his mid-80s and still healthy, could not conceal his disappointment. My poor wife fretted and nagged. I felt worthless. I know now I had all the classic signs of clinical depression. I slept a lot. I just couldn't get moving. I was living life in a disconnected slow motion.

I got defensive when my wife suggested I see a psychiatrist. What an admission of weakness, to see a head mechanic. A shrink! But my wife made it clear. Get some help or we're through. I tried one counselor and didn't feel comfortable at all. The second guy I saw was OK. He came across like a regular guy. We had some great talks, and I got a lot off my chest. He gave me some pills, too, which made a huge difference in my outlook. I'm on the wagon now. Not a drop. Go to AA regularly. I want to take this opportunity to thank my wife for giving me the kick in the rear I needed and for sticking it out with me. Invincible? Not me. Just human.

Computer scientist — Jamestown, N.Y.

Points to ponder

- Once you leave a job and are out of the loop, you are quickly forgotten. These are rules one and two.

- Chemical dependency can sneak up on you during times of distress. When friends and professionals want to help, let them.

- There is no such thing as job security, so don't put all your self-esteem eggs in the vocation basket. Cultivate a life outside of work.

Alzheimer's disease and why diagnosis requires ruling out other causes of the symptoms, such as strokes and brain tumors.

Examination under a microscope of the brain tissue of someone who had Alzheimer's reveals pathologic changes known as plaques and tangles. Plaques are dense deposits of protein and cellular material that form outside and around the brain's nerve cells (neurons). Tangles are twisted fibers that build up inside the neurons.

Plaques, which consist largely of the protein beta amyloid, first develop in the part of the brain used for memory and other cognitive functions. They form 10 to 20 years before symptoms appear. Tangles are mainly made up of the protein tau.

Researchers don't yet understand the role of plaques and tangles in Alzheimer's disease. They suspect that both of them cause neurons to degenerate, lose their ability to communicate and die, leading to an irreversible loss of brain function.

How likely are you to get Alzheimer's disease? No one knows for sure. Age certainly is a factor. Among people 65 years old, one or two in 100 have Alzheimer's. It rarely affects those younger than age 40, but early-onset Alzheimer's is considered a different form of the disease. The average age of diagnosis is about 80. By that age the risk increases to one in five. Half of all people who live to age 90 have symptoms.

Heredity plays a role in about 40 percent of people with early-onset Alzheimer's. There's also increased risk of later-onset Alzheimer's if it's in your family, but even in families that have several members who develop the disease, most people don't get it. Researchers are still studying its causes.

Research brings hope. As disheartening as the prospect of getting Alzheimer's disease is, thanks to research, exciting advances are being made in treatment. Here's a look at some of the most promising:

- *Acetylcholine inhibitors.* The neurotransmitter (a chemical that bridges gaps, or synapses, between neurons) acetylcholine drops up to 90 percent in people with Alzheimer's disease. Three drugs, tacrine (Cognex), donepezil (Aricept) and, most recently, rivastigmine (Exelon), block the breakdown of the neurotransmitter in an effort to slow cognitive decline. The drugs seem to help slow the disease, at least for a time, in 30 percent to 50 percent of people with mild to moderate symptoms.

- *Estrogen replacement therapy.* The longest and largest study of estrogen replacement therapy (ERT) to date, published in 1999 in the *Journal of the American Medical Association (JAMA),* found that ERT had no significant effect on the course of Alzheimer's once the disease was diagnosed. But a 16-year study of 472 women, sponsored by the National Institute on Aging (NIA), indicated that ERT may reduce the risk of developing the disease. Until more research is completed, however, prevention of Alzheimer's isn't enough of a reason to take ERT.

- *Vitamin E.* Vitamin E is an antioxidant that counters the damage caused to cells through oxidation. In high doses it may help to prevent the brain cell damage of Alzheimer's. A study published in the *New England Journal of Medicine,* in which Mayo Clinic participated, showed some promise in vitamin E's ability to slow the progression of the disease. Further studies are needed. Also being studied is selegiline (Eldepryl), an antioxidant used to treat Parkinson's disease.

- *Ginkgo.* Ginkgo comes from the Ginkgo biloba tree. It is an herb long used in China as a remedy for a number of ailments, and it has been touted as a memory aid. A study published in *JAMA* and a review of research published in the *Archives of Neurology* suggest that the herb may stabilize or improve the quality of life for some people with Alzheimer's. A federally funded study tracking 2,000 healthy 75-year-olds was launched last year to determine whether ginkgo can delay the onset of Alzheimer's and other dementias.

- *Nonsteroidal anti-inflammatory drugs and corticosteroids.* Inflammation in the brain may play a role in Alzheimer's. Some research has indicated that use of nonsteroidal anti-inflammatory drugs (NSAIDs), such as ibuprofen, or corticosteroids, such as prednisone, may decrease the risk of developing Alzheimer's. Newer medications called Cox-2 inhibitors may be an option for prevention or stabilization of Alzheimer's disease in the near future.

- *Nasal vaccine.* Researchers are studying the idea of a nasal vaccine for Alzheimer's. It has only been tested in mice, but a snort of synthetic beta amyloid peptide reduced plaques in the mice's brains, according to a study published last year in the *Annals of Neurology.*

Researchers also are coming closer to being able to diagnose Alzheimer's without a brain biopsy. These tools show promise:

- *Structural magnetic resonance imaging.* Research published in the *Annals of Neurology* demonstrated that by using structural magnetic resonance imaging (MRI) to measure the volume of certain brain regions affected by Alzheimer's, researchers could predict with high accuracy who would get the disease, even before clinical signs appeared. As new treatments are developed, early identification of people at high risk of the disease could prove critical to treatment efforts.

- *Genetics.* Researchers have identified genetic mutations that cause early forms of Alzheimer's (onset before age 60). Although there's no evidence that these genetic mutations cause the more common, age-related form of Alzheimer's, genetics do play a role in it. In particular, a gene known as apolipoprotein E (APOE) seems to play a role in developing age-related Alzheimer's. Eventually, genetic testing could lead to early diagnosis of the disease.

Numerous clinical trials are being conducted for Alzheimer's disease, so if you or a loved one has been diagnosed with the disease, talk to your doctor about participating in one. Whether you or a loved one has the disease or you just dread the possibility of getting it, it's important to remember that researchers are making progress and there's hope for the future.

For more information, log on to our home page and search on the word *Alzheimer's.* Here's our Web site address: *www.MayoClinic.com.*

Also try the Web site of the NIA's Alzheimer's Disease Education and Referral Center: *www.alzheimers.org.*

Messing with your mind

As mentioned earlier, alcohol, nicotine and drugs, whether prescription or illegal, can cause or contribute to anxiety and depression. They're addictive substances, which research indicates change brain chemistry. They also affect your health and diminish the quality of your life. Obviously, illegal drugs, such as marijuana, cocaine and heroine, can destroy your health and your life. But did you know that even caffeine, that most popular of addictive substances, can mess with your mind? Here's how:

Caffeine. Numerous studies have been done on the effects on your health of caffeine, one of about 500 chemicals in coffee. Most of the studies are inconclusive, partly because so many variables are involved in coffee processing and consumption. The type of bean, the degree of roasting, the method of brewing and what you add to your coffee all influence the chemical composition of what you end up drinking. It also doesn't help research efforts that coffee drinkers are more likely to be older, to smoke, to drink more alcohol and to eat poorly, so research, for the most part, hasn't been able to separate the effects of caffeine from other factors.

As a result it's hard to determine how much coffee you can consume safely. There's no doubt, however, that caffeine is a stimulant that affects your brain. It can wake you up, give you energy, make you more alert and speed up your reaction time. It can (depending on your sensitivity) raise your blood pressure, speed up your heart, cause or worsen heartburn, interrupt your sleep and cause anxiety. Caffeine can make you irritable and restless and worsen panic attacks. That nerve jangling, jumpy feeling you get after you've had too many cups of java isn't your imagination. Caffeine also can create dependence. Just try quitting cold turkey. That nasty headache indicates withdrawal.

The average American adult consumes about 200 milligrams of caffeine a day, which is enough to make some people feel anxious.

A living fossil

As the first female manager of my company, I had to prove myself every day. I had broken through the glass ceiling and was now running with the boys, the Big Dogs as they say. I had finally arrived, or so I thought. I always assumed my people skills and connections would sail me smoothly into retirement. But I was blindsided by technology.

With little transition or time to adjust, our company entered the e-commerce era. Every division in every location went online. Information services and marketing spoke a new language. We were no longer a company, but a "B-2-B enterprise." Decisions had to be made about "customer relationship management" software and capital outlays for "enterprise resource planning." Of course I learned the new jargon, but behind the words was technology with which I was completely unfamiliar.

I felt like a grandmother, surrounded by young computer savvy kids talking fast about database management, data matching, cleansing and mining. Please just give me an overhead projector and a piece of chalk! I knew how to word process and send e-mail, but I still preferred my IBM Selectric.

Of course a manager makes decisions and relies on staff to possess technical skills to carry out those decisions. That was true up to a point. But even a manager must have a big picture grasp of fundamentals. I didn't. I felt like a living fossil.

I was 57 at the time and had hoped to stay on until 65 to maximize my pension. But the writing was on the computer screen. They "groomed" me for early retirement. The new manager is half my age, a woman who never had to claw her way to the top like I did. She didn't even know my name.

Communications manager — St. Louis, Mo.

Points to ponder

- Keep your skills up-to-date so that changes in your profession do not take you by surprise.
- Be nimble. Anticipate changes, and be flexible enough to reinvent yourself periodically.

About three-fourths of that comes from coffee. The rest is in carbonated beverages, teas, chocolate, cocoa, over-the-counter (OTC) pain relievers and products designed to help you stay awake.

As far as your health is concerned, you can do without caffeine quite nicely. But if you like caffeinated coffee, cola or tea, then consume them in moderation. If you want to cut down or quit, then do so gradually to avoid the headache, fatigue and other symptoms that can accompany withdrawal.

Alcohol. Talk about murky areas. You've undoubtedly heard about the studies that show the beneficial effects of moderate alcohol consumption on your heart. Does that mean you should take up drinking? The answer is no. If you don't drink, then don't start.

Unfortunately, the disease often referred to as alcoholism is a serious problem among older adults, many of whom don't begin drinking heavily until their 60s or 70s. Heavy drinking can be a way of responding to a major life change, such as the death of a spouse, divorce or retirement. More women than men take up drinking later in life. Alcoholism may be undetected until major health consequences show up.

Too much alcohol (more than one drink a day for women or more than two a day for men) can harm almost every organ and system in your body. It increases the risk of cardiovascular disease, liver and pancreas disease, sexual dysfunction and some cancers. It also weakens the immune system, leaving you more vulnerable to infections.

As you age, your body is less able to handle alcohol, so it takes less to do damage. And alcohol abuse can help speed the aging process along. A study presented at the American Academy of Addiction Psychiatry indicated that alcohol abuse may cause what looks like the physical signs of aging, including falls and insomnia.

Another study found that anxiety disorders go hand in hand with alcohol abuse. The risk of having anxiety is three times greater if alcohol abuse is present, although no one is sure why. It could be that being anxious makes some people drink or, as noted earlier, that drinking makes some people anxious. It could also be that genetic or environmental factors predispose certain people to both anxiety disorders and alcohol abuse.

In a study published in the *American Journal of Drug and Alcohol Abuse*, of adults age 65 and older who were seen in an emergency room, those who drank heavily tended to perceive their health as worse in the year following their visit. In addition, heavy drinking can complicate older people's health conditions by causing adverse interactions with drugs, noncompliance with diet or medication directions, cognitive impairment and psychiatric illness. It can also create health problems such as hypertension and gastric bleeding.

Alcohol clearly affects your cognitive abilities and your concentration. If you enjoy a glass of wine with dinner, then there's probably no reason to give it up. But if you find yourself drinking more or if you turn to alcohol for comfort, then you may have a problem. That's especially true if you can't cut down or quit, despite your best intentions. Talk to your doctor about treatment options.

Nicotine. There's nothing good to say about nicotine. If you smoke or chew tobacco, then do your best to quit. It's never too late, and the longer you go without nicotine, the more damage you can reverse, even if you've used it for years.

With one puff on a cigarette, you take in 4,000 chemicals. Nicotine is the one that hooks you. It's so addictive, it's harder to kick than heroine or cocaine. When you inhale the smoke, nicotine goes to your brain within 10 seconds. If you smoke a pipe or a cigar (the smoke of which most people don't inhale) or chew tobacco, the nicotine gets absorbed somewhat more slowly through the mucous membranes of your mouth.

Once nicotine reaches your brain, it increases the neurotransmitter dopamine, which regulates movement, emotion, motivation and, most important for the addictive process, pleasure. The acute effects of nicotine dissipate almost as quickly as they strike, which means you have to keep taking in more to keep the pleasurable feelings going.

Because nicotine is so addictive, quitting smoking is hard. If you're a former smoker, quitting may be one of the hardest things you've ever done. If you want to quit, it may be the hardest thing you ever will do. Withdrawal symptoms can last a month or more and can include irritability, craving, difficulty thinking and paying attention, sleep disturbances and increased appetite. But there is help. Nicotine replacement products, such as gum, inhalers, nasal sprays and skin patches, behavioral therapy and the antidepressant bupropion (Zyban, Wellbutrin) have proven effective in helping people quit.

Think of the alternative. Smoking has been linked to high blood pressure, gum disease, heart disease and a variety of cancers, particularly but not exclusively lung cancer, as well as other lung diseases. Every year, smoking cigarettes causes one in five deaths in this country. Smoking won't just mess with your mind — it's likely to kill you. If you're a smoker and healthy aging is your goal, then you must quit. For more information on nicotine dependence, see our Web site at *www.MayoClinic.com* and search on the word *nicotine*.

Medications. If you're like most people, chances are you're taking more medications, both prescription and OTC, than you did when you were younger. Unfortunately, some of the most common drugs can cause symptoms similar to those of dementia, including confusion and memory loss. The problem is compounded not only by taking more than one medication but also by your metabolism, which becomes less efficient as you age.

Drugs also can interact with food and vitamin and mineral supplements. To avoid such problems, do the following:

- Make sure your doctors are aware of everything you take, including OTC medications, herbs, vitamins and minerals.

- Read all of the directions, warnings and precautions for all of the drugs and supplements that you want to take.

- Tell your doctor about any side effects you experience.

- Take medications as directed. If they are to be swallowed, take them with a full glass of water. Take them with food if indicated.

- Don't stir medications into food, mix it into hot beverages or take it with vitamin and mineral supplements.

- Don't break time-release capsules without first talking to a pharmacist — breaking them may destroy the time-release.

Abuse of medications can cause you serious problems. If you find yourself unable to go without certain medications, such as sleeping pills, pain relievers or tranquilizers, or if you need to keep taking more of the drug to get the same effect, talk to your doctor.

About your memory

Remember when you were in grade school and you had to memorize big chunks of information, such as all of the state capitals or the words to the poem "The Midnight Ride of Paul Revere"? If you think you were able to do that then only because of your youth, think again. You were able to do it because you worked hard at committing the information to memory. When was the last time you did that? Chances are if you tried it now, you'd be as successful as you were then.

Think of your memory as being divided into three parts. Here's how it works:

Working memory. You look up a phone number in the yellow pages, maybe repeat it to yourself until you can get to the phone to dial it. Then, poof, it's gone. Chances are if you have to call the same number again later, you'll have to look it up. Your working memory stored it only for as long as you needed it.

Short-term memory. Your short-term memory is where you store more important information or information that you're exposed to frequently. It stays there for hours or even days. Do you remember what you had for breakfast this morning? That's your short-term memory at work.

Long-term memory. Information that's really important, like your daughter's birthday or the words to an oft-repeated prayer, or something that has an emotional impact, is in your long-term memory, where it may be stored for years. Working at committing

Memory muscle

I'd always prided myself in having a good memory. As a schoolgirl, I seemed to memorize and retain facts and figures easier than so many of my classmates. You can imagine how worried I was when my memory began to slip. I began to forget things, little things for the most part — items for the grocery list or the name of a person I was just introduced to a few minutes ago. Sometimes details of what I had just read or been told did not stay with me. Or I'd forget what I was doing before being interrupted. Car keys. Glasses. Stuff like that.

I shared my concern with friends. "Join the club," they said. "It's happening to us all." But I was concerned that what was happening to me was not normal. My mother spent her final years with dementia. It might have been Alzheimer's, but back then they weren't calling it that.

I talked to my doctor, who thankfully took my concerns seriously. She gave me some tests and a physical and could find no medical problems. I'm not on any medication that affects memory. She then referred me to a clinic that tested my attention span, visual memory and reading retention. They tested how well I could remember a list of numbers, as well as faces and names.

I scored well, they told me. Perhaps I had lost some memory ability over the years, but my memory was still quite good, and I did not have any kind of dementia. I told them I was still bothered by the change. They explained that we can all improve our memories by using simple techniques of association and repetition and by improving our concentration. They gave me a book of exercises to improve memory.

I think it has helped. I find that associating a name with an object, for example, is particularly helpful. Just being more aware of how memory works helped me sharpen mine. I make lists. I put my keys and glasses in the same spot when I get home. I am just fine, thank you.

Homemaker — Corpus Christi, Texas

Points to ponder

- Some forgetfulness is a normal part of aging, not a precursor to Alzheimer's.
- Memory exercises and recall techniques can improve your memory.

something to memory helps it move into long-term storage. For example, if you worked hard at memorizing "The Midnight Ride of Paul Revere" as a child, chances are you can recall at least a few lines of the poem even now. The repetition helped lock it in.

Neurotransmitters and neurons play a role in embedding your memories, although researchers don't know for sure how the process works. What they do know is that neurotransmitters tend to decrease with age, so your ability to retrieve information is likely to be slower than it was when you were younger.

That doesn't mean that it's inevitable your memory will falter as you get older. Oh, sure, you'll probably forget where you put your glasses. You probably did that in your 20s, too, but then you were more likely to laugh it off because it didn't scare you and you didn't see it as a sign of old age.

If you find yourself forgetting things, here are some things you can do to aid your memory:

Tips on remembering. Take a lesson from those long-ago days when you were forced to commit certain facts to memory. If it's important for you to remember something, then work at it. Here's how:

- *Repetition.* Practice saying something over and over, and chances are it will be yours forever.

- *Associations.* Create a story, make up a rhyme or link new information to something you already know, such as the words to a song. That will help lodge the information in your brain.

- *Breaking it down.* Break information down into small pieces and learn it bit by bit.

- *Visualizations.* Create an image in your brain that you associate with what you're trying to remember. When you are introduced to someone, remember his or her name by thinking of a visual cue related to it. Also repeat his or her name as you shake hands.

Keep in mind that memorizing is hard work. You might want to save the effort for what's really important. For other information, try keeping lists or placing reminders in places where you'll come across them, such as on your bathroom mirror or refrigerator door. Keep a calendar. Make a habit of putting things you use regularly, such as your glasses or your car keys, in the same place every time so that you'll know where they are. When you park your car, make note of what aisle you're in. If it's not marked, count the number of aisles from a certain spot, such as a door or a signpost. Write it down, if necessary. Or say it out loud. If you park on the unmarked second floor of a parking ramp, think of a baseball double-header, or form a victory V with two fingers. That will help you remember.

Mind and matter

If you're not depressed or anxious, if you don't have Alzheimer's disease or another form of dementia, and if you haven't suffered a brain injury, such as from a stroke or an accident, you can keep your memory in tiptop shape by taking good care of yourself. Specifically, you can:

- *Eat well.* Earlier in this chapter, you read about vitamin E's potential to slow the progress of Alzheimer's disease. It may be that vitamin E and other antioxidants (particularly vitamins A and C), which help counter the damage to cells caused by oxidation, may aid memory in general. They certainly contribute to your good health, which is important for keeping your mind functioning at its best. So eat your veggies. And fruits. And whole grains. Keep saturated fats to a minimum. If you drink alcohol, do so in moderation.

- *Keep moving.* Physical activity, like eating well, contributes to overall health. Besides countering depression, it can help lower blood pressure and combat stress, all of which can affect your mind. Select activities you enjoy and try for 30 minutes of low to moderately intense physical activity daily. You can break it up into 10- or 15-minute sessions and still reap the benefits.

- *Manage your stress.* When you're under stress, your body cranks out high levels of the stress hormone cortisol. According to a study in the *Archives of General Psychiatry*, high levels of cortisol can interfere with your ability to remember words, phone numbers and other details. You can't avoid stressful events, but you can control how you react to them. Keep a positive attitude. If you need help, talk to friends, join a support group or seek professional help.

- *Maintain social contacts and keep active.* Most importantly, keep your mind active. Take classes, learn a new skill, pick up a foreign language, take up the violin, play chess, work crossword puzzles, read a book, volunteer. Limit television watching. Challenge your grandkids to a game of Scrabble. Remember, lifelong learning is key to keeping your mind fit.

For more information, log on to our home page and select the Food and Nutrition Center. Here's our Web site address: *www.MayoClinic.com.*

Chapter 4

Your spirit

Take-home messages

- **Be aware of the broader picture.**
- **You are more than tissue and chemicals.**
- **A belief system can give order and purpose to life's changes.**

L ife is change, and the longer you live the more change you're likely to encounter. Change is challenging, even if you think the change being made is for the better. Sometimes change challenges you profoundly, even shaking you to your roots. Loss of a loved one, retirement, moving to a new community or becoming ill can be such a change.

How do you deal with change? What gives you strength in difficult times? What bolsters you and keeps you steady when it feels as though the earth is shifting beneath your feet?

For many people the answer is their faith. That faith encompasses not only a belief in a higher power and an order to the universe, but also connection to others. It's those connections that keep people stable when life's ever-shifting winds threaten to blow them off course.

Once upon a time, healers understood the link between people's spirits and their well-being. Health and spirit were inextricably linked. In many cultures, priests and shamans were the healers, and they enlisted their charges' spirits to restore their wholeness.

As science ascended in the 19th and 20th centuries, however, modern medical techniques nudged aside faith's role in healing. Yet even the miraculous medical discoveries of the last century didn't push faith out of the picture entirely. Think of all the medical centers, such as Mayo Clinic, that were founded as part of a religious order throughout the 20th century.

From its earliest days, Mayo Clinic was associated with the Sisters of St. Francis. Spirituality was so important to the Mayo brothers that even while struggling with the financial difficulties brought on by the Great Depression, Dr. William J. Mayo insisted that the need for money was not to override the importance of spirituality.

"The maintenance of the present spiritual status of the Mayo Clinic is of the greatest importance," Dr. Mayo told the faculty of the medical school. "We must not permit the material side to encroach upon our ideals. ... I believe the heart of the Clinic has been more responsible for its extraordinary usefulness to the people and the confidence that the people have in it than any other factor."

With the upsurge of things spiritual in this country over the last decade or so, practitioners of modern medicine are reconsidering the connection between faith and healing. "It's becoming clear that medicine and religion are entering a new dynamic of mutual respect and inquiry. There is a convergence — not a collision — and it will determine the future of health care," Virginia Harris, chairwoman of the board of the entity that publishes the *Christian Science Monitor*, recently told a gathering of health care practitioners.

Faith factors into health and, therefore, into healthy aging. More and more studies are indicating that when you believe in something larger than yourself, you strengthen your ability to cope with whatever life hands you.

In this chapter we'll look at the powerful effects of spirituality on aging. If you don't think of yourself as religious, you may be tempted to skip this chapter. Please don't. We're talking about spirit, not religious affiliation. You may be surprised to learn of the varied and often surprising forms in which spirituality expresses itself, and of the ways it can help you cope with life's inevitable transitions.

New interest in spirituality

You only have to browse a bookstore or flip through magazines to know there's a rise in spirituality in this country. In fact, surveys show that more than 50 percent of Americans pray daily. And more than 80 percent of 1,004 Americans polled toward the end of the 20th century said they believed in the healing power of prayer.

For most people, spirituality or faith — believing in that spiritual something larger than yourself — contributes to good health. Study after study shows that people who attend religious services (service attendance is easier to measure and classify than people's beliefs) enjoy better health, live longer and recover from illness faster and with fewer complications. They also tend to cope better with illness and experience less depression.

For example, one study found that the blood pressure of older adults who attended religious services at least once a week and prayed or studied the Bible at least daily was consistently lower than the blood pressure of those who engaged in religious activity infrequently or not at all. Another study found that the more religious participants reported being, the faster they reported recovering from depression, compared with those who were described as less religious.

Among those who are seriously ill, many use their spiritual beliefs to cope with their illness. Of more than 850 studies that have examined the relationship between religious involvement and various aspects of mental health, more than two-thirds have found that people adapt to stress better if they're religious. In a study of 108 women with breast cancer, 93 percent indicated their beliefs helped them sustain their hope.

Those are just some of the numerous studies that have attempted to measure the effect of religious belief on illness and recovery. In reviewing many of those studies, researchers at Georgetown University School of Medicine found that at least 80 percent of the studies suggested religious belief has a beneficial effect on health. The researchers concluded that religious factors are associated with increased survival; reduced alcohol, cigarette and drug use; reduced anxiety, depression and anger; lower blood pressure; and improved quality of life for people with cancer and heart disease.

No one knows exactly how faith or spiritual belief and practice affect health. Some experts attribute the healing effect to hope, which has been shown to benefit your immune system. Others liken prayer to meditation, which decreases muscle tension and lowers heart rate. Still others point to the social connectedness, another healing factor that regular worship attendance fosters.

The research on faith and health also has its detractors. Critics point out that those who are more religious also are more likely to practice good health habits, such as reduced alcohol, cigarette and drug use. Clearly, there's more to maintaining good health than just spiritual belief. Yet you can't dismiss spirituality's contributions. An editorial in the *Journal of the American Medical Association (JAMA)* stated, "Research on religious factors in health is as sophisticated as any other growth area within epidemiology, and, given the topic, findings have often been subject to even greater scrutiny."

Ultimately, though, does it matter what the research shows? You can't acquire faith because you think it will contribute to healthy aging. And you're not likely to lose it even if you were to find out tomorrow that it offers no health benefits whatsoever. Faith stands on its own.

There is enough evidence, however, to suggest that faith can help you live a longer, healthier life. Even if it doesn't lengthen your life, it can strengthen your ability to cope, and thereby improve the quality of your life. If that weren't so, why would 72 of the 125 undergraduate medical schools in the United States, including Mayo Medical School, teach courses on spirituality and healing? In the mid-1990s, only three medical schools offered such courses.

Citing all the evidence in support of the health benefits of spirituality, the *Annals of Internal Medicine* urged doctors to respect the spiritual needs of the people they treat, especially if they hope to get the best results from whatever treatment they prescribe. Science is beginning to validate what many people have known intuitively all along: When it comes to healthy aging, your faith is working in your favor.

But what, exactly, is spirituality?

As noted previously, many of the studies on religion and health have focused on worship attendance. For instance, in a study published in the *American Journal of Public Health*, more than 2,000 people age 55 and older were followed for 5 years. Those who reported regular (at least weekly) attendance at religious services were less likely to die during the 5-year period than those who didn't. The study took into account other variables, such as health status at the outset, health habits and social support.

But faith isn't restricted to those who belong to an organized faith tradition, and the effects of faith on health aren't limited to improving mortality. Perhaps more important is faith's role in improving your quality of life and increasing your resilience.

What if you're not part of an organized tradition? That doesn't mean you're not spiritual. People often use the word *spirituality* interchangeably with religion, but the terms aren't the same. Religion has more to do with following the practices and dictates of an institution. Spirituality is more personal and individual and encompasses your relationships with others and with your Creator.

The Spirituality in Healthcare Committee at Mayo Clinic offers the following definition: "Spirituality is a dynamic process by which one discovers inner wisdom and vitality that give meaning and purpose to all life events and relationships."

According to a clinically tested scale of spiritual well-being, spirituality can include any or all of the following: belief in a power greater than oneself, purpose in life, faith, trust in divine guidance, prayer, meditation, group worship, ability to forgive, ability to find meaning in suffering and gratitude for life.

"Spirituality as a dynamic process helps individuals discover meaning and purpose in their lives, even in the midst of personal tragedy, crisis, stress, illness, pain and suffering," says a report of Mayo's Spirituality in Healthcare Committee. "This process is an inner quest. This quest involves openness to the promptings of one's soul or spirit, silence, contemplation, meditation, prayer, inner dialogue and/or discernment. Spirituality empowers a person to be fully engaged in life experiences from birth to death."

Being fully engaged in life includes being connected — to others, to a higher power, to community and to the natural world.

Your spirituality may be the one thing that can't be taken from you. While imprisoned in the Nazi concentration camp Auschwitz during World War II, psychiatrist Viktor Frankl found meaning in the most extreme suffering. Cut off from his family, stripped of his possessions and subjected to brutality, hunger and cold, he discovered that spirituality helped him and others rise above their circumstances. In *Man's Search for Meaning*, he writes:

> In spite of all the enforced physical and mental primitiveness of life in a concentration camp, it was possible for spiritual life to deepen. Sensitive people who were used to a rich intellectual life may have suffered much pain…, but the damage to their inner selves was less. They were able to retreat from their terrible surroundings to a life of inner riches and spiritual freedom. Only in this way can one explain the apparent paradox that some prisoners of a less hardy make-up often seemed to survive camp life better than did those of a robust nature.

In Frankl's experience, faith sustained a prisoner; loss of it doomed him. Frankl writes, "With his loss of belief in the future, he also lost his spiritual hold; he let himself decline and became subject to mental and physical decay."

Frankl isn't talking about religion or even about God specifically. He's talking about faith, a belief in the existence of an ultimate purpose. It helped him and many other prisoners survive Auschwitz, arguably the most devastating and demoralizing of experiences, with their spirits intact.

That being the case, think of what your faith can do for you. When faced with some of life's greatest challenges, such as the death of a spouse, the loss of your life's work (as in retirement), disability or illness, your spirituality can sustain you and help you heal.

Keep in mind, though, that healing doesn't mean curing. Rather, healing can mean achieving serenity by accepting yourself as you are, coping with whatever life brings and living the best life you can despite your losses. Sometimes healing is of the soul, not of the body.

"When you come to the edge of all the light you know, and are about to step off into the darkness of the unknown, faith is knowing one of two things will happen," says writer Barbara Winter. "There will be something solid to stand on, or you will be taught how to fly."

Other aspects of spirituality

We've seen how Viktor Frankl's ability to find meaning in suffering helped sustain him in Auschwitz. Let's look at some of the other aspects of spirituality — including hope, forgiveness, meditation, helping others, gratitude, social connectedness, and prayer and ritual — that can help sustain you through the challenges of aging.

Hope

"I must reluctantly observe that two causes, the abbreviation of time, and the failure of hope, will always tinge with a browner shade the evening of life," wrote English historian Edward Gibbon in the 1700s. In other words, toward the end of our lives, as we run short of time, loss of hope can rob us of the richness of our lives.

Hope is as old as humankind. So is despair. Hope mitigates the darkness. Could you survive, much less thrive, without it? Hope can play a crucial role in the quality of your life if you're facing a crisis, such as diagnosis of a chronic disease or loss of a loved one.

In *The Power of Hope: The One Essential of Life and Love*, Rabbi Maurice Lamm writes, "But we now know that hope can … make us better able to manage daily stresses and setbacks. It can help us ride out severe personal crises and cope with critical illness. It can even enable us to enhance the way we handle our own aging, and to be more satisfied with life."

Despite all the despair that life sends our way, he writes, hope wins. But sometimes it fades and needs a jump-start. "Regenerating our hope often requires an explicit, conscious effort — especially when it looks like it's slipping away in the twilight of our lives," he writes. "We have spent all our lives in hope, and we should not be willing to surrender so easily."

Forgiveness

Think of someone who has hurt you. The hurt can be a minor insult (someone pushed ahead of you in line at the grocery store) or something extremely painful (a drunk driver killed a loved one). What do you feel when you think about the offender?

Chances are you feel angry, hostile and vengeful. Your blood pressure might be rising, your heart pounding. Now that you've filled your mind and body with these thoughts and feelings, it could take you a while to be able to focus on anything else. You've surrendered

A sense of belonging

My wife died of ovarian cancer at age 41. I was never socially outgoing, which made coping with Joanne's death harder, I'm sure. By my late 40s, I decided to jump-start my life and pull out of my cynical funk.

Since I was 5 years old, I'd wanted to act in plays. But I was too shy. In high school, a friend tried to pull me onto the stage to audition, but I yanked my arm away and ran. Then time passed quickly with work, marriage and kids.

I saw a newspaper ad for acting lessons at the community theater. Halfway up the creaky stairs to the rehearsal room, I did an about-face and started to leave. No, I told myself. You will do this. I forced myself to go up.

The bug bit. I studied my practice parts. I read *An Actor Prepares* and *Audition*. I showed up for every class. I had not felt so good about things in a long time. Two weeks after the classes ended, the director who taught them asked me to play one of the servant's in Molière's *The Miser*. Not long thereafter, at age 52, I played Scrooge.

A Christmas Carol embodied all I love about theater. We had a large cast of all ages and backgrounds. Young and old mingled without barriers that sometimes separate the ages. Backstage, the Cratchit kids and street urchins scampered, sometimes teasing old Ebenezer and pretending they were frightened of me. Marley bored your serenity and well-being to the person who hurt you or to the event. Does it feel good to be in this state?

Mind-body experts believe that harboring vengeful and painful feelings toward someone who has hurt you puts your body under ongoing stress. In fact, a number of studies have shown the heart-damaging effects of hostility. Other studies indicate that holding on to anger may increase your risk of developing high blood pressure, as well as damaging your emotional health. So what do you do? You try to forgive.

us all with his obsession with railroad history trivia. Teenagers in the cast flirted. Station in life was irrelevant. The corporate chairwoman was glad to be part of our happy group.

Fezziwig, Mr. and Mrs. Cratchit, the Portly Gentlemen and the rest of us elders made new friends and laughed more than we had for a long time. Cast or crew, it didn't matter. We were a family, creating enjoyment for others. When we walked through that backstage door for rehearsal and stomped the snow off our boots, the day's troubles melted away. We all shared tremendous humor and energy. What a thrill.

Outside is the big world. Sometimes our little world of theater reflects the big world, so we can understand it better. The irony of Scrooge's transformation and its similarity to my own did not escape me. When I'm in a play, I'm living in the moment. It's a feeling of being alive, of belonging and, yes, of love. Shakespeare was right: "All the world is a stage, and we are actors."

Amateur actor — Northampton, Mass.

Points to ponder

- Doing something creative with others can energize and uplift you spiritually.
- Go with your gut and pursue your dreams.
- You only go around once. Be willing to take chances.

Forgiving someone who has hurt you could be one of the hardest things you ever do. First, you need to understand what forgiving isn't. It isn't forgetting, denying, condoning or excusing. It is dropping the burden of your anger and resentment and foregoing revenge. It's refusing to let the painful feelings consume you. It's realizing that forgiveness is a lifelong process that you'll probably need to revisit many times throughout your life. But even if you've been carrying a grudge a long time, it's never too late to forgive.

Researchers at the University of Wisconsin have been studying forgiveness for more than a decade. They've developed a model of forgiveness that involves four phases:

First, you acknowledge your pain.

Next, you recognize that something has to change if you're to heal. You entertain the possibility of forgiveness, then commit to forgiving.

Then comes the work phase, the really hard part. You strive to find a new way of thinking about the person who hurt you and learn to accept the pain of your experience. In doing so, you may develop empathy and possibly even compassion for the person who hurt you.

In the last phase, you begin to realize that you're getting emotional and possibly spiritual relief from the process of forgiving.

The process may or may not lead to reconciliation with the one who hurt you. But forgiving lessens your pain, helps you move forward and may add deeper meaning to your life.

Meditation

If there's one thing that mind-body medical studies have determined, it's that meditation can be beneficial to your health. Its effects include lowering heart rate, blood pressure and cholesterol, controlling stress, and easing anxiety and chronic pain.

If meditating conjures up images of twisting yourself into a pretzel and chanting unfamiliar words, then you should know that meditation takes many forms. Almost every belief system embraces meditation.

Meditating is really pretty simple and straightforward. It can be religious, but it doesn't have to be. Some people meditate to get closer to their higher power. Others do it to relax and clear their minds. Whatever your motivation, meditation can be good for you.

Two elements are necessary for meditating: something to focus on, such as your breath or the repetition of a word, thought, sound or prayer, and an ability to bring yourself gently back to your focus when other thoughts intrude, which they definitely will.

Want to try it? Find a quiet place where you won't be interrupted. Get into a comfortable position. Sit on a chair or a cushion on the floor. You can even lie on your back. But don't get too comfortable because you don't want to fall asleep. Decide how long you want to meditate and stick with the time, even if you feel bored or restless. You can start with 5 or 10 minutes. Keep a clock or watch nearby and peek at it from time to time. Don't set an alarm because the sound would be jarring.

Pick a focus. It can be your breathing, or you can choose a prayer, word or phrase to repeat over and over. Or you can count to four over and over, timing the count to your breathing (two counts for each in breath, two counts for each out breath). Whatever you choose, be prepared to stick with it for several weeks before trying something else.

The hard part about meditation is that it takes dedication and practice. Do it every day, even if only for 5 minutes. Do it even if it feels like you're wasting your time. Don't worry if you can't calm your mind. You're not doing it wrong. Just keep coming back to your focus every time your mind wanders.

Try to be patient and don't expect dramatic results. If you stick with it, then you're likely to discover the ability to calm yourself in stressful situations. You may be better able to brush off life's little annoyances, such as waiting in long lines. Eventually, your practice may result in health improvements, such as lower blood pressure.

If you think you can't meditate, then think again. "Thinking you are unable to meditate is a little like thinking you are unable to breathe, or to concentrate or relax," writes Jon Kabat-Zinn, Ph.D., one of the pioneers of using meditation to improve health. "Pretty much anybody can breath easily. And under the right circumstances, pretty much anybody can concentrate, anybody can relax."

Helping others

With rare exception, everyone wants to feel productive. What would make you feel older than feeling useless? So what do you do when you're ready to give up your job, or retirement takes it from you, especially if you derive much of your identity and feelings of productivity from your work?

One way is to volunteer. Nearly 14 million people over age 65 serve as mentors, counselors, reading teachers, crime victim advocates, school and library aides, drivers for social service agencies, helpers at hospitals and nursing centers, and care providers for people who are homebound.

Giving your time and talents to a worthwhile cause can offer you a number of benefits. Besides making you feel productive, it can boost your self-esteem, help you develop new skills and make you feel more connected to your community. Some studies even suggest that volunteering can boost your health and help you live longer. You never know what doors may open as a result of your giving of yourself.

In the previously mentioned study in the *American Journal of Public Health*, which showed that people who attended religious services weekly tended to live longer than those who didn't, volunteering upped their chances of a long life even further.

If you'd like to volunteer but don't know how to get started, then talk to someone at your place of worship or a local hospital, jail, school or community network. If you have a passion for a particular cause, such as mentoring youth or helping people who can't read or write, then look for local or national organizations that provide the type of services you'd like to participate in. Or contact charitable organizations for information.

Gratitude

It's so easy to take good things for granted and to focus on what's wrong. That's especially true if you have a chronic illness or disability or other potentially overwhelming circumstance. But focusing on what's wrong can wring the last drop of joy from your life.

Everyone has something to be grateful for. Most people have many reasons for gratitude. If you make a habit of noticing and giving thanks, then your attitude eventually will brighten, and life will look better.

Try this: Every night before you go to bed, think of five things that happened that day that you're grateful for. They can be as simple as a beautiful sunset or as profound as recovery from cancer. Say thanks to your Creator, to the universe or to someone who made your life a little better.

Brother David Steindl-Rast, author of *Gratefulness: The Heart of Prayer*, writes: "As I express my gratitude, I become more deeply aware of it. And the greater my awareness, the greater my need to express it. What happens here is a spiraling ascent, a process of growth in ever-expanding circles around a steady center."

Social connectedness
Possibly one of the reasons attendance at worship services is so healthy is that it provides those who attend with a social network. A number of studies have shown that belonging to a strong social network may increase longevity and that having support from others may protect you from the destructive effects of stress and boost your immune system. In the words of Bette Midler, "Ya gotta have friends."

Research indicates that people who have no social network are under more stress and live shorter lives than those with social ties. In fact, their chances of getting sick and dying early are double those of people who get by with a little help from their friends. Friends and family who offer a shoulder to cry on help you cope with problems and avoid depression. And having people who care about you may motivate you to take better care of yourself.

Your social network doesn't have to be large. It's not how many friends you have that matters, but the quality of your relationships with them. If you're giving more than you're getting, then the relationships may be more draining than nurturing. You need at least one person who nurtures you as much as you nurture him or her.

If you have good relationships, then make an effort to feed them. Stay in touch. Let friends know you're thinking of them by dropping a card, sending an e-mail or making a phone call. Consider reconciling with those with whom you've had a rift. Say you're sorry and forgive. Make new friends by reaching out to others. Invite them to join you for coffee or a meal. Let them know you want to get to know them better.

If you find yourself alone and disconnected, don't despair. There are ways to reach out to others. Try some of these avenues:

Check out your senior center. It's a good place to find companionship, as well as food and activities. If transportation is a problem, ask whether the center provides a shuttle service, or find out whether your community offers a transportation service for seniors.

Get active in your faith community. Attend services, participate in programs, take classes, volunteer to lead a discussion group in which you can share expertise you developed in your life, your career or your hobbies.

Take a class. Your local college, junior college or university might offer something you've always wanted to learn. But don't limit yourself. You may find courses in unexpected places, such as at a public garden, museum or library, or on the Internet.

Join an exercise class or walking group. You'll improve your health in more ways than one.

Investigate the Elderhostel programs. Find one in a place you've always wanted to explore and make plans to visit.

Join a support group. If you have a chronic illness or have suffered a loss, then chances are there's a support group for you. In such a setting you can share your feelings with others who are having similar experiences. Besides offering emotional support, groups provide information and keep you from feeling socially isolated. To find a group that's right for you, ask health care professionals, hospitals, your place of worship or an organization, such as the American Cancer Society, the American Heart Association or the Arthritis Foundation, that specializes in the issues you're dealing with.

Prayer and ritual

The expression, "There are no atheists in foxholes," reminds us that in times of crisis, most people ask for help. Prayer brings comfort, helps you form a connection with your higher power, gives you an avenue for expressing gratitude and sustains you through difficult times.

Prayer has such power that some studies have shown that intercessory prayer, having strangers pray for one who's sick, may aid healing. Many faith communities offer prayers for those who are ill. However, more studies are needed before any real conclusions can be drawn about intercessory prayer.

Ritual helps bring order to your world. "Through rituals," writes Rabbi Debra Orenstein, "we create structures that provide an element of predictability and, therefore, safety around times of insecurity, transition and/or loss."

Even if you don't realize it, you have rituals in your life. A yearly ritual could be something as basic as buying your grandkids new shoes before they start school every fall. Think about what that does for you and for them. Besides bringing a sense of security to what is often a chaotic world, rituals can strengthen your bond with family, friends or community.

Prayer and ritual can help you deal with losses and keep you centered when the ground seems to be shifting beneath you. That's why most faith traditions have established rituals for life's most difficult transitions, such as the death of a loved one. For other times, such as divorce, completing menopause or learning you have a chronic illness, there may be no established rituals in your tradition. But that doesn't mean you can't create your own. Just as you can pray either by reading from a book or by speaking from your heart, you can follow established rituals or make up your own for any of life's transitions.

Whatever your spiritual expression, whether it be your connection to nature or your connection to your faith community, whether you pray or meditate or drink in the sunset every day, it can nourish you. Your spirit can increase your resilience and help you cope with life's changes, give you a better sense of yourself, help you choose faith over despair in your darkest times, and provide a sense of order and stability during periods of chaos and crisis.

Of her own spiritual journey, Anne Lamott writes in *Traveling Mercies: Some Thoughts on Faith*:

> My coming to faith did not start with a leap but rather a series of staggers from what seemed like one safe place to another. Like lily pads, round and green, these places summoned, then held me up while I grew. Each prepared me for the next leaf on which I would land, and in this way I moved across the swamp of doubt and fear. ... Each step brought me closer to the verdant pad of faith on which I somehow stay afloat today.

Your finances

- **No one has a greater stake in your finances than you.**
- **Be proactive when it comes to financial planning.**
- **Many options are available. Get help if you need it.**
- **Financial security is tied to health.**

Money isn't everything, the old saying goes. And indeed it isn't. For most of us, family, faith, career and other concerns rank higher. But money is one of the resources we need to make our way in the world. It helps to determine whether we live comfortably — whatever that means for us individually. It allows us to do the things we want to do with the new free time we suddenly have at our disposal in retirement. Not least, it helps us to help others and to make a difference in the communities we live in. In short, money gives us options. It opens doors.

To not have enough money can make retired life difficult and frustrating. In fact, not having adequate financial resources can be a major stress on your emotions and, ultimately, on your health. People with good finances consistently cope with illness better than people who don't have the funds they need. In other words, having the money to live a comfortable, interesting retirement is important for your well-being — along with good nutrition, a healthy emotional, spiritual and social life, exercise and seeing your doctor regularly.

Achieving a financially secure retirement, however, is largely an individual's responsibility. The buck stops with us. The days of retired workers being taken care of entirely by old-fashioned company pensions and Social Security benefits are long past. We're now largely responsible for planning our own retirements.

Government statistics show that the current generation of retirees has planned well. The median net worth of households headed by people age 65 or older increased 69 percent between 1984 and 1999. Today's future retirees, however, won't necessarily enjoy the same level of security unless they act now to achieve their retirement dreams.

Without good planning and discipline, there's no guarantee that your retirement income will cover your expenses, let alone allow you to fulfill your hopes for retirement. If you haven't started already, a good way to begin is to look at how much money you think you'll need and compare it with how much money you're likely to have. If you come up short, it may not be too late to take steps toward making up the difference.

How much money will you need?

The fact that you're going to retire doesn't mean that bills will stop arriving in your mailbox. It doesn't mean that you will suddenly lose your desire to travel, eat in good restaurants or have season tickets for pro football. It doesn't mean that your leaking roof won't require replacement. The money you need or want isn't apt to change much from the days you were collecting your paychecks. You might even require more, depending on your plans. Some experts suggest that we need 80 percent of our preretirement gross income after we retire. Others maintain that we require 100 percent of what we made during our working life.

It's up to you to determine how much money you'll need to support a retirement lifestyle you're comfortable with. To do that you'll first want to consider how long you're likely to live. A well-reasoned view of your potential life span can help you avoid the problem of outliving your financial resources.

Estimate your life expectancy

Of course, all of us want to live as long as possible and stay as healthy and active as we can. It's only natural to desire many, many more years with our loved ones, our friends, our interests, our causes. But you might ask, not unreasonably, "How do I know how long I'll live? I could live to be 100. Or a truck could run me over tomorrow."

In general, the average 65-year-old American man today can expect to live to 81. An American woman the same age can expect to live to 84. But you're a unique individual, not an "average" American. To plan for your retired years, you need to look at your own health history, your lifestyle, your family history and other factors to arrive at the most likely number of years between retirement and the end of your life.

Scientists who specialize in human aging believe that three factors are key to predicting how long a person is likely to live:

• Heredity

• Lifestyle

• Environment

The health and life expectancy of your parents and grandparents can be a predictor of how you're likely to do. If they all lived to a ripe old age, the odds are that you will, too. However, if something like heart disease, cancer or neurologic illness runs in the family, you might not need as big of a retirement fund.

How you choose to live has a huge effect on how long you live. If you eat too much, gain excessive weight and don't exercise, you're asking for trouble — such as diabetes, heart disease or cancer. If you drink too much alcohol, use tobacco or take recreational drugs, you increase your chances of dying younger. But if you stay active, have social connections, keep your weight at a reasonable level, avoid tobacco use and drink moderately, you help your chances of living longer and healthier.

Where you live and work also can affect your life expectancy. For example, if you live in a place with environmental pollution or inadequate sanitary conditions, you may be exposed to greater risk of getting ill and dying younger. If you work in a dangerous job or in a dangerous environment, your odds of a long life may be reduced.

No one can accurately predict how long you'll live, but researchers do know that certain factors influence life expectancy. To see how you measure up, calculate your life expectancy at the Web site *www.livingto100.com.*

Decide when you'll retire

The age at which you retire will have a big impact on how much money you'll have for retirement. By working longer you'll have more time to put money away into retirement accounts. In addition, you won't be drawing money out of your retirement accounts as soon, allowing them to continue growing through interest and dividend accumulations. This is especially important for tax-deferred investments. Resist the urge to withdraw funds as long as possible so that they continue to grow.

To see how your retirement age will affect your Social Security benefits, take a look at "Your Social Security Statement," which the Social Security Administration is required to send you each year. Under the benefits section, you'll find figures showing how much your monthly payment will be if you retire at age 62, age 66 or age 70. Find the difference between your payment if you retire at 62 and your payment if you retire at 70. Now multiply this difference by 12 months and then by the number of years you hope to live after retirement. You'll understand why waiting to retire can be a smart financial move.

There are good reasons for choosing to retire at a younger age. Maybe you are in poor health. Maybe you don't want to work any longer, and you have enough money to retire early. In any case it's smart to ask your tax adviser when it's best for you to start drawing Social Security. To estimate your personal Social Security benefits, see the Web site *www.ssa.gov/mystatement/ssst2.htm.*

Calculate your expenses

In addition to gauging how many years you're likely to have after retirement, you need to make a realistic estimate of how much you're likely to spend. Experts generally believe that the average retiree should plan on having between 80 percent and 100 percent of his or her yearly gross preretirement income. Once again, though, you are not an average retiree. You're a unique individual whose needs may or may not fit some norm.

You may find after retirement that you need more money than you did immediately before retirement because you suddenly find yourself free to do the things you love, full time. Perhaps you'll travel extensively. Perhaps you'll need to purchase equipment for some long-deferred hobby. Maybe you'll move to a warm climate where it costs more to live.

Later in your retirement you may need some assistance to get along, at home or in a care setting. Moreover, your medical expenses will almost certainly increase.

In between — after you've gotten those retirement wild oats out of your system but before you require extra services — you may well settle down and live quite inexpensively, by choice. During this time you might downsize your living arrangements and spend time instead of money, doing things like taking care of grandchildren and volunteering at the local museum.

The point is to clearly assess your own plans and hopes. Then — if you haven't done so as a matter of course — keep track of your current spending habits. Add up all — yes, all — expenses for a few months to see where the money goes. Compare that against hypothetical budgets for your early, middle and later retirement years.

You may find that the retirement money you're slated to receive — based on your current estimates of all sources of income — won't be enough to finance the trips you want to take or that second home in a warm climate. In fact, it might be inadequate to support your current lifestyle. Fortunately, there still may be time to beef up your retirement resources — by saving more now.

Alternatively, you can make plans for a less ambitious retirement — reducing your standard of living. Maybe retiring at a younger age is more important to you than beefing up your retirement funds. For many people it's a fair trade: less money but more time to enjoy retirement.

Perhaps your retirement goals are more modest in the first place, as befits your frugal personality. You have every intention of staying close to the home you've paid off, doing some golfing, reading stacks of mystery novels and tackling some volunteer work around town. In that case a relatively modest retirement nest egg may be big enough for you.

Many retirees choose to keep working to some degree — either in their chosen fields or in some new career. They may do it as a practical matter, to produce the extra income they feel they need during retirement. Or they may do it because they enjoy keeping active and engaged in the workforce. As of January 2000, anyone who has reached his or her full retirement age (currently age 65) can earn unlimited income without losing Social Security benefits. And that can help support a solvent, successful retirement. If you are a working retiree under your full retirement age, you will lose benefits if you make more than the annual limit, which is currently $10,680.

It's important, in any event, not to assume that you have — or don't have — enough money for retirement. You need to take a hard look at the following:

- Your current spending habits
- Your anticipated retirement income
- Your plans for your retirement years and their prospective costs

Then factor in all of the living expenses that come your way, whether or not you are retired, from insurance and property taxes to utilities and college tuition. And don't forget the potential extra costs of getting old — bigger medical expenses, living assistance, home care and long-term care.

Then you'll have an idea of the kind of money you're likely to need after you walk out of that retirement party at your workplace. However, there's another vital money question you need to consider before celebrating: How much will your money be worth?

The American Savings Education Council has created a simple worksheet to estimate how much money you'll need by the time you retire to maintain your current standard of living. You'll find the Ballpark Estimate Worksheet at *www.asec.org*.

How much will your money be worth?

You probably know how much money you have right now in accounts earmarked for retirement. But is it possible to calculate how much that money will be worth by the time you retire in 10, 15 or 20 years? You can get a pretty good idea by starting with this thought: The higher the interest rate you receive on your money and the longer your money is allowed to grow, the bigger your account will be by the time you retire.

The benefits of compound interest

Value over time of $1 invested once at various interest rates

Interest rate*	Years						
	5	10	15	20	25	30	35
4%	1.22	1.48	1.80	2.19	2.67	3.24	4.80
6%	1.34	1.79	2.40	3.21	4.29	5.75	10.29
8%	1.47	2.16	3.17	4.66	6.85	10.06	21.72
10%	1.61	2.59	4.18	6.73	10.84	17.45	45.26
12%	1.76	3.11	5.47	9.65	17.45	29.96	93.05

*Interest compounded annually

The rule of 72 and the joy of compounding

A common equation for figuring out how long it will take your retirement investments to double is the Rule of 72. This equation states that 72 divided by the interest rate you receive equals the number of years it will take for your money to double. (This assumes you are reinvesting your interest or dividends into your account.) For example, a money market fund with an average annual interest rate of 6 percent will double your money in 12 years. A mutual fund that consistently offers 10 percent growth a year will double in 7.2 years.

One factor that helps your money grow faster is compound interest. With simple interest you receive interest on only the amount of your initial deposit or investment. For example, if you deposited $1,000 in an account that paid 6 percent simple interest annually, each year you would earn $60 on the account.

With compound interest you receive interest on the initial deposit and on the interest that accumulates in the account. So in our example, in the second year you would receive 6 percent interest on $1,060, or $63.60. In the third year you would earn $67.42 interest. Over a period of years, the compounding advantage can add up to a great deal of money. In addition, interest can be compounded annually, semiannually, quarterly or even more frequently. The more frequent it is compounded, the faster your money will grow.

Unfortunately, it's difficult to predict the behavior of two well-known economic forces that nibble away at all our investments, robbing them of a certain amount of value over the years — inflation and taxes. As you make financial plans for your retirement, think about not only how much money you'll have when you retire but also what that money will be worth in real terms.

Inflation eats it up

Remember when gas was 20 cents a gallon and bread was 40 cents a loaf? Did you pay more for your last car than you paid for your first house? Inflation occurs when the price you pay for goods and services rises and doesn't come back down. You pay more than a dollar for the same services and goods a dollar used to buy. Your money is worth less.

The U.S. government gauges the rate of inflation with a statistical measure called the Consumer Price Index (CPI), which keeps track of the changes in price of 400 common goods and services. Some prices go up, some go down, but the general trend is toward inflation.

In any case inflation is not a constant. Though it has remained at relatively low and manageable levels in recent years, a generation

The buying power of $100 over time

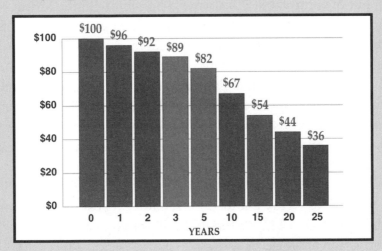

How inflation can affect your savings

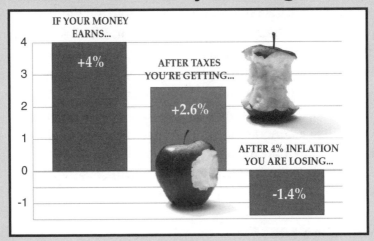

Is saving money the same as investing money?

If you answered no, you realize that saving money may maintain your original dollar deposits — your principal — but it won't go far in creating financial gain on that. The interest earnings on your savings are unlikley to keep pace with inflation.

Saving money is not the same as investing money. Key differences include higher interest rates available with investment products, such as mutual funds and stocks, and the compounding effect of these higher interest rates. These factors give you a better opportunity to outpace the erosion of inflation. In financial planning terms, saving money may help maintain your set-aside dollars, while investing may help you achieve income growth.

The chart above illustrates how inflation can affect your savings, assuming an inflation rate of 4 percent and a tax rate of 36 percent.

ago it was quite high. There's no immediate prospect of inflation getting out of control, but it's always a possibility in the future. High inflation is considered to be among the most destructive of economic forces, one that economists, federal regulators and bankers work hard to keep at bay.

But whether inflation is high or low, it tends to accumulate and deplete the value of money over the course of years. That means that certain items you buy today will cost a little bit more a year from now and much more when you retire. For instance, if you bought a soda in 1955, it probably cost you a nickel or a dime. Today it'll cost you a buck. If you bought an ordinary automobile in the early 1960s — say a four-door sedan — it cost somewhere in the neighborhood of $2,000. Today it will set you back $20,000. That's inflation at work.

Anyone who made retirement plans in the 1960s for the year 2000 and budgeted $2,000 for a new car in 2001 would be in trouble. Anyone who remembers a hospital stay in the '70s costing only $60 a day would be in for a shock entering the hospital these days.

The same thing may happen to the goods and services you'll need or want in retirement, assuming retirement's not in the near future. The $20,000 automobile of today could well become a $100,000 vehicle a generation in the future. That's why it may be dangerous to think that the retirement figures you arrive at today — which are adequate for today's costs — will cover what you need in the future.

Taxes still take a bite

"In this world nothing is certain but death and taxes," wrote Benjamin Franklin in 1789. Although a lot has changed since then, his words of wisdom hold true. No one knows how much the tax rate will go up or down, but you can bet that you'll still be paying something in taxes when you retire. And if you've managed to acquire a big enough nest egg, the income you derive from it may put you in a higher tax bracket than you're in now. Don't expect that just because you're an honored retiree and senior citizen the Internal Revenue Service is willing to overlook the taxable income you receive. In addition, you probably will have paid off your mortgage by the time you retire, and that means you'll have less to deduct from your taxable income.

The retirement calculator at *www.money.com* takes you through some basic steps to gauge whether the money you're putting away now will support you during retirement. The calculations factor in variables such as goals, inflation and annual returns on investments.

Sources of income

Your retirement income will probably come from a combination of sources. These are likely to include Social Security, savings and investments, retirement funds and pensions, and earned income.

Social Security

When President Franklin Roosevelt signed the Social Security Act into law in 1935, it was an acknowledgment that working Americans and their spouses deserved financial security as they grew older, regardless of their economic status. For over six decades Americans of retirement age have relied to some degree or other on their monthly Social Security payment.

In its earlier days, the monthly Social Security payment was almost enough to support a retired American. But as the decades have proceeded, that check has become less and less adequate to the task of supporting an individual retiree in a reasonable manner. The average retired worker receives only 43 percent of his or her preretirement income as Social Security. If you earn $65,000 annually, your benefits will equal only 24 percent of your preretirement income. If you earn a higher income — say $200,000 — Social Security will replace only 8 percent of it.

Yet Social Security remains the most important income for nearly two-thirds of Americans 65 or older. For 25 percent of that group, it provides 90 percent of their income. Needless to say, retirees who rely largely on Social Security will enjoy relatively sparse incomes during their "golden years." Or they'll have to continue working.

On the plus side, Social Security is portable — no matter how many jobs you've held, it travels with you right to the end of your working days. And it's largely insulated against the forces of inflation by a cost of living adjustment (COLA).

The operative description, though, is *largely*. The COLA is based on a component of the Consumer Price Index called the CPI-W, which reflects inflation for hourly and urban clerical workers, not older adults. For nearly two decades the CPI-W has noted inflation of 3.1 percent, while the component pegged to Americans 62 and older, the CPI-E, has reflected inflation at 3.5 percent. This means that for older adults, even the Social Security COLA doesn't quite keep up with inflation.

By all accounts, Social Security will be able to handle the demands of the baby boom generation until about 2030. After that it may not be able to provide full benefits. Changes may need to be made to keep the system financially healthy. Benefits may be reduced, or the age at which you can access them may go up. Workers may have to pay more into the system. The amount you receive may be based more on need than entitlement, with well-to-do retirees getting no benefits at all. Workers may be given the option of putting their Social Security dollars into investments such as stocks and bonds.

Whatever happens, the wise retirement planner understands that Social Security ought to be merely a single component in a multipronged scheme to fulfill the financial needs of his or her retirement years. That's why you need to gain an understanding of the part that Social Security will play in your retirement income. By seeing clearly where Social Security fits in your retirement plan, you can proceed to compensate for its prospective deficiencies with other sources of income.

"How much Social Security am I entitled to?" The amount of Social Security benefit you get at retirement depends on the amount of Social Security taxes you pay during your working years. To receive the maximum benefit, you need to have worked for 35 years at or beyond the maximum taxable salary for each of those years. If you've worked part time throughout your career or held lower paying jobs, you can expect to receive substantially less.

No matter how far along you are in your working years, you can find out approximately how much Social Security benefit you're likely to receive by requesting a statement of how much you've earned over your career. You can call the Social Security Administration (SSA) at 800-772-1213 and ask for a form SSA-7004, or you can download it from the SSA Web site at *www.ssa.gov.* When you receive the form, you'll be asked to provide information such as your Social Security number, your earnings for last year, your expected earnings for the current year and an estimate of future average yearly earnings. If you're doing a retirement plan with a spouse or a partner, have him or her request a form as well.

In a few weeks you'll get back a statement that provides you with:

- A history of your earnings
- Your Social Security contributions over the years
- An estimate of your retirement benefit (depending on when you retire)
- Your benefit if you were to become disabled
- The benefits your spouse and minor children would get should you die

Keep in mind that these figures can vary. Your income could go down or up — either planned or unplanned. Congress could institute changes in Social Security benefits. You'll only know for sure what your benefits are after you apply for them.

"When should I start collecting Social Security?" The age at which you apply for Social Security locks in the amount of your monthly benefits. If you apply at 62, your benefits will be about 20 percent lower than if you had waited until 65. If you're a 62-year-old on Social Security, that 20 percent lower benefit is permanent and the benefit will not increase at age 65 except for annual COLA adjustments. You need to balance the temptations of an earlier retirement against a potential two or three decades of lower benefits.

Until the spring of 2000, many would-be retirees who planned on continuing to work had a very good reason not to take Social Security at the full retirement age of 65: If they kept working, they had to return one dollar's worth of Social Security benefits for every three dollars' worth of earned income over $17,000. But a new law allows working retirees to earn as much as they're able to after age 65 and still collect their full Social Security benefits. However, as of 2000, if you retire between the ages of 62 and 64, you'll have to return one dollar for every two dollars you earn over the annual limit of $10,080.

Poverty among older adults

The net worth of many older Americans has increased in recent years. But 10 percent of those age 55 and older still live in poverty. Two-thirds of that group are women, and that figure increases as age goes up. This is because women live longer than men and because many older women spent time at home raising families and did not, therefore, earn full-time incomes or earned at a lower rate than men. This means they didn't build up as much money in retirement funds and Social Security benefits. According to the Women's Institute for a Secure Retirement, the pension benefits of retired women are half those of their male counterparts.

Older women living in poverty are more likely to be single or members of a minority. In 1998, 47 percent of divorced black women between 65 and 74 lived in poverty.

Social Security is of vital importance to the poorest among older adults. For those older people in the lowest two-fifths of the income brackets, Social Security constitutes 80 percent of their income.

If your retirement plan makes it feasible to delay your Social Security benefits beyond age 65, you can earn what's called delayed retirement credits (DRCs). For each year you delay collecting benefits, your benefits will increase between 3 percent and 8 percent, depending on your age. Taking DRCs would prove a good choice only if you live for a long time after 70. And there's no way of guaranteeing that eventuality. The bottom line is, seek advice from an expert on when to start collecting your Social Security benefits.

For help with your retirement planning, check out the SSA's Web site at *www.ssa.gov*. You'll find answers to frequently asked questions, useful planning guides and the most current information on Social Security benefits.

Savings and investments

If it weren't for the erosion caused to our retirement nest eggs by inflation and taxes, many of us might not be inclined to accept much risk in our investments. If we could count on a steady 5 percent to 8 percent interest in safe, fixed-income investments such as savings accounts, certificates of deposit (CDs) and bonds of various kinds, we could build our retirement funds with little fear of risk.

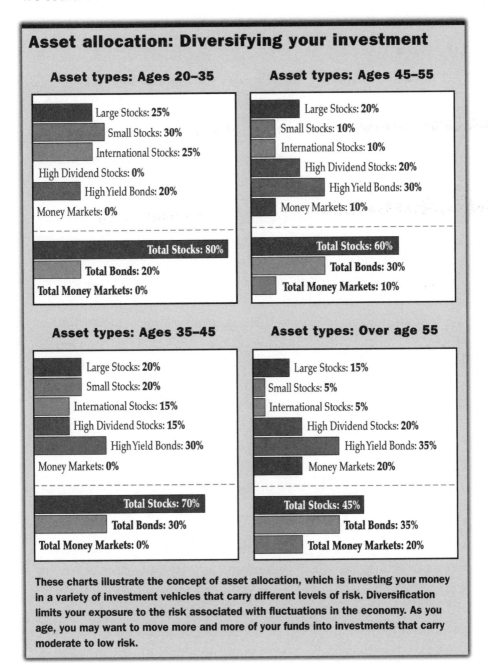

Asset allocation: Diversifying your investment

Asset types: Ages 20–35

Large Stocks: **25%**
Small Stocks: **30%**
International Stocks: **25%**
High Dividend Stocks: **0%**
High Yield Bonds: **20%**
Money Markets: **0%**

Total Stocks: **80%**
Total Bonds: **20%**
Total Money Markets: **0%**

Asset types: Ages 45–55

Large Stocks: **20%**
Small Stocks: **10%**
International Stocks: **10%**
High Dividend Stocks: **20%**
High Yield Bonds: **30%**
Money Markets: **10%**

Total Stocks: **60%**
Total Bonds: **30%**
Total Money Markets: **10%**

Asset types: Ages 35–45

Large Stocks: **20%**
Small Stocks: **20%**
International Stocks: **15%**
High Dividend Stocks: **15%**
High Yield Bonds: **30%**
Money Markets: **0%**

Total Stocks: **70%**
Total Bonds: **30%**
Total Money Markets: **0%**

Asset types: Over age 55

Large Stocks: **15%**
Small Stocks: **5%**
International Stocks: **5%**
High Dividend Stocks: **20%**
High Yield Bonds: **35%**
Money Markets: **20%**

Total Stocks: **45%**
Total Bonds: **35%**
Total Money Markets: **20%**

These charts illustrate the concept of asset allocation, which is investing your money in a variety of investment vehicles that carry different levels of risk. Diversification limits your exposure to the risk associated with fluctuations in the economy. As you age, you may want to move more and more of your funds into investments that carry moderate to low risk.

But in the real world, inflation and taxes could consume up to half of the value of your hard-earned retirement dollar in such safe investments. And that may be motivation to seek out investments that offer greater prospective rewards. But, of course, with greater potential rewards comes greater potential risk.

Whatever you choose to do, your tolerance for risk is a very personal thing. Some of us can stand very little risk and prefer to take our chances primarily with safe but low-yielding investments. Others may be inclined to gamble and go with high-risk stocks or other speculative equities. Most of us fall somewhere in between, balancing risk and security. Where you stand in this range of personalities will help determine your investment mix at various stages in your preretirement life.

In general, the younger you are the better equipped you are to accept risk and sustain the loss that it can bring. As you get closer to retirement, you'll want to decrease risk in your investment portfolio. You'll want more investments that provide reliable income rather than appreciation in value.

Early in your career, if you have a high tolerance for risk, you might consider putting up to three-quarters of your money into stocks and stock mutual funds, with the balance in fixed-income investments such as CDs and bonds. If your risk tolerance is low, you might put only a third into stocks and stock mutual funds, and the balance in fixed-income investments such as CDs and bonds.

As an investor who's worried about risk and getting on toward retirement, you might reduce your stock and mutual fund holdings by 20 percent or 30 percent and increase your fixed-income investments.

If you think you'd be very uncomfortable losing money or failing to make any money at all — as even solid equity stocks sometimes do — you probably have a low tolerance for risk. If, however, you're not rattled by drops in your stocks' value or lack of performance over the short term — and understand that effective investing in stocks takes a long view — you can consider yourself fairly risk tolerant. Just remember, your retirement may last 30 years, so you ought to plan for adequate sources of income over a long run. Whatever you decide, be true to your own level of risk aversion.

Savings accounts. Unless you're fortunate enough to have a wealthy aunt or uncle planning to leave you a large bequest, chances are you'll need to save money from your paycheck to fund the retirement investment strategy you'd like to follow. For most Americans the first stop for much of that money is in a bank or credit union account. These accounts tend not to do much for growing your retirement dollar — with minimal interest rates that barely keep up with inflation — but they're very safe, and they generally make your money easy to withdraw. Think of them as parking lots for your cash, and not a long-term solution.

- *Savings accounts.* A basic savings account allows you to add and remove money from your account at your discretion. Savings accounts pay a small amount of interest on the account balance. Many savings accounts require a minimum balance.

- *Checking accounts.* A basic checking account allows deposits whenever you want. You take money out of the account by writing a check or using a debit card or cash card. Some checking accounts also pay a small amount of interest on your balance, much like a savings account. Many checking accounts have minimum required deposits and other terms and conditions. You may have to pay fees if you don't meet those terms and conditions.

- *Money market deposit accounts.* A money market deposit account is a lot like a checking account, but with a higher minimum balance. It usually pays a higher rate of interest than an ordinary interest-paying checking account.

- *Certificates of deposit.* Certificates of deposit (CDs) provide you with better interest rates than any of the other savings accounts. The upside of CDs is that these rates are locked in for the term of the CD — anywhere from a few days to several years. The downside is that if you want to get your money out of a CD before its term is finished, you may have to pay the bank a penalty, and you pay taxes on the interest earned each year, even if it is simply accruing on the CD and not actually paid to you.

Bonds. There are two ways to participate in the big, capitalist world beyond your own job or your own business: By buying equity, or shares, in companies (more on equity below), or by buying debt issued by companies and governments that promise to pay you back with interest in a specified number of months or years. These debt instruments are usually called bonds. They appeal to many investors because of their general reliability and low risk. Many different types of bonds are available — they are offered by governments, governmental agencies and corporations:

- *U.S. treasury bills.* U.S. treasury bills (T-bills) are widely considered the safest investment you can own. You buy them directly from the U.S. Federal Reserve Bank (*www.publicdebt.treas.gov*) for a minimum of $1,000. The interest is credited to you immediately, and you get your principal back at the end of the bill's term — 3, 6 or 12 months. Interest is free of local and state taxes.

- *U.S. treasury notes.* U.S. treasury notes (T-notes) have terms of 2 to 10 years but pay your interest semiannually rather than up front. They can be bought directly — like T-bills. You can sell them on the open market, if you wish to, and make extra money if the going rate has dropped lower than the interest rate you're receiving on them.

- *U.S. treasury bonds.* U.S. treasury bonds are like T-notes, except they have longer maturities — 10 to 30 years.

- *Municipal bonds.* Municipal bonds are debt instruments offered by governments of various kinds — states, counties, cities. They're always exempt from federal taxes and may be state tax exempt, unless they originate outside your state of residence. In that case you pay state tax. You'll need to invest a minimum of $5,000, and you'll be able to choose from among various maturities — short-, medium- and long-term.

- *Corporate bonds.* Corporate bonds require a minimum $5,000 investment as well. They may pay a higher interest rate than government bonds, but they also represent more risk. In a sense corporate bonds resemble stocks — they're only as good as the financial strength of the company issuing them. Buy them with the same care as you would buy individual stocks.

• *High-yield or junk bonds.* These bonds are government or corporate bonds from entities with relatively low credit ratings. They offer a higher yield because they are higher risk investments.

Bonds are rated according to their level of risk by two leading services — Standard & Poor's and Moody's. A Standard & Poor's rating of AAA (Aaa for Moody's) is the top rating (the lowest risk bond). Bonds with ratings of AA or A are still quite good but riskier than bonds rated AAA. BBB bonds may be a decent investment but do entail some risk. Any bond with a rating of BB or lower (down to D) is considered a junk bond. Junk bonds may offer higher yields, but they are considered quite risky. Only invest in junk bonds if your risk tolerance is high and you don't mind losing some money.

Stocks. Of all investments, stocks — shares of ownership in corporations — have the greatest potential to reward and to punish. If, for instance, you had invested in leading Internet companies in the mid-90s and sold your stocks before the so-called dot.coms took a beating in 2000, you might have made very large gains. But if you had held onto them into 2000, they could have lost much of their value. At any given time that you decide to sell your stock, it could have made you good money, made you no money at all or lost you money.

Fortunately, you have a broad spectrum of stocks to choose from. The two basic classes of stock are preferred and common.

Preferred stock is for those who want regular, specified dividend income from their investment and the security of having a higher claim than common stockholders do on the assets of the company, in case it's liquidated. With preferred stock you are not allowed to vote at shareholders' meetings and may not be given other rights available to owners of common stock.

If you opt to buy common stock, you have the right to vote at shareholders' meetings or by proxy (a kind of absentee ballot). You get to participate in the election of the directors of the company. You get to buy newly created shares of stock before any nonstockholders. But you won't necessarily get dividends, and you're last in the queue for receiving any money if the company is liquidated.

In terms of market capitalization (or market cap), which means the total value of all of a company's stock, stocks come in three sizes: small cap, mid cap and large cap. Small caps are small, sometimes volatile companies that usually seek to grow aggressively, with a market cap of up to $1 billion. Mid caps combine growth and stability, with values between $1 billion and $10 billion. Large caps have values over $10 billion and tend to offer stability, some growth potential and good dividends. AT&T and IBM are examples of large caps.

Among the thousands of stocks available to American investors, there are several categories.

- Blue chip stocks represent large, well-known corporations with solid histories of rewarding investors with reasonable growth and dividends. They're among the least risky of stocks. Only 30 of the top blue chips make up the Dow Jones industrial average.

- Growth stocks are stocks of a company that's intent on growing its earnings above all else and generally pays no dividends. It tends to be riskier than blue chips and other large caps, but with the potential of greater appreciation.

- Income stocks provide less growth but greater-than-average dividends. If you're close to retirement or retired, income stocks can help provide you with a steady income stream.

- Value stocks are stocks of essentially sound companies with solid earnings but low share prices. In other words they're more valuable than their price indicates — potential bargains.

You can also choose among stocks by market sector, such as high tech, biotech, financial, health care, insurance, media, utilities, transportation and energy.

Stocks have the potential to be very rewarding for your retirement nest egg. But given their ability to also punish, they're no place for an inexperienced investor. Before you put your retirement-bound dollars into a stock, you need to either thoroughly research it yourself or work with a broker or investment counselor whom you trust.

Mutual funds. Even if you'd like to participate in the stock market as a part of your retirement investment plan, you may not be comfortable with buying individual stocks — either because you don't trust your judgment in picking stocks or because you don't have a broker or a financial adviser who meets your requirements. Or it may simply be that you do not want to put too many eggs in one basket (one company, or one type of stock).

In any of those cases, stock mutual funds may be the answer. Stock mutual funds own dozens, hundreds, or even thousands of individual company stocks. These funds offer the investor the opportunity to own shares in many companies. The investment philosophy of the fund may reflect the personal judgment of a fund manager. In that case the mutual fund would probably have a general approach or philosophy that the manager would do his or her best to execute successfully — such as achieving growth, providing income or investing in certain market segments (such as energy, biotech or financial).

There are two types of mutual funds: load and no-load. A "load" is a sales charge payable to a broker or to the fund, or to both. Given the quality and performance of today's no-load funds, there's little reason to buy a loaded fund.

Like stocks, stock mutual funds come with different levels of risk.

- Equity income funds generally invest in stocks that provide good dividends, such as utilities and blue chips. They have a moderate level of risk.

- Growth and income funds seek to offer solid dividends while having the value of the stocks they own grow. They're also at a moderate level of risk.

- Stock index funds mirror how specific markets and indexes perform. For example, you could buy a fund that replicates the Standard & Poor's 500 index, containing all 500 of those selected stocks. Index funds tend to have a moderate level of risk.

- Large-cap funds are made up of stocks from the largest, best-established corporations. They're considered somewhat less risky.

Tuning your financial engine

Such a short time ago we were newlyweds with little babies and a big mortgage. Now the house is paid for, and the youngest of our three is about to graduate from college. We were still 20 years from retirement when I started to worry about our financial picture, simply because the picture wasn't clear to me.

My husband was confident we were on course to retire comfortably. We are what you'd call comfortably middle class, maybe even upper middle class. But how did we know we'd have enough money for retirement? Were we making the smartest decisions on how to handle our money? After all, we could live to be 100.

An ad on TV prompted me to suggest to my husband that we consult with a financial planner. In the ad, all of these well-to-do looking people with seemingly nothing to be concerned about were secretly worried they didn't have their financial house in order. I felt like one of those people. Our financial picture was so fragmented. My husband had pensions waiting for him at two of his former employers as well as where he is now. I have a 403(b) at a local college where I still teach English literature. Add to that our miscellaneous IRAs, 401(k)s, mutual funds, stocks, life insurance and an online trading account with an Internet broker. We needed help sorting this out.

My husband bristled a bit at the implication it was more than he could handle. He likes to bike, so I smoothed his feathers with an analogy he'd appreciate. Our finances, I told him, are like spokes on a bicycle wheel. If one's broken, the rest aren't going to work as well as they should.

We asked friends for names and found a young man who immediately impressed us. He charged a flat hourly fee and did not represent any line of financial products, so he wasn't trying to sell us anything. He was a fee-only planner.

He gave our finances a complete physical exam. We learned we were doing OK, but we weren't as financially healthy as we hoped to be. For starters, he suggested a slight shift in investment strategy that would save some taxes. He showed us how, in our circumstance, it makes more sense to take my husband's defined benefit pensions in a lump sum and invest them in an IRA, instead of getting monthly payments from an annuity. He also showed us a couple ways we could do a better job of protecting our estate from taxes. And we talked about trusts so that all our hard-earned money would not be wiped out by taxes.

Then he put all our financial information on computer and made us a "financial biography," a notebook that contained everything we and our children need to know about our insurance policies, retirement funds, trusts, wills and estate.

He helped us save a lot of money, much more than what he charged. We were surprised at what can be done that most people aren't aware of. We even talked to him about my mother's possible need for long-term care. He knew the latest rules for retaining assets if you have to pay for nursing home care. He assigned power of attorney in case she becomes incapacitated and helped us decipher the jargon in a long-term-care insurance policy we were considering.

Now my husband likes to tell friends that financial planning is like fixing a car. There was a time when you tuned your own, but electronic ignition makes that impractical. Today it takes a specialist to pop the hood and see if your financial engine is tuned. No one has a greater stake in your financial well-being than you.

College instructor — Philadelphia, Pa.

Points to ponder

- Wise financial planning is too important an issue to be left to chance.

- A good financial planner can help you manage your assets and live comfortably during the 20 or more years you may live after retirement.

- Financial planning is more complicated than it used to be because you have more investment options.

- A good financial planner does not take control of your finances but, instead, keeps you in control.

- Mid-cap funds have holdings in medium-sized companies. While they offer better potential returns than large-cap funds, they come with higher risk.

- Growth funds go for robust earnings growth only, but may not do well when the market drops. They have higher risk.

- International funds own shares in foreign companies and represent higher risk.

- Aggressive growth funds offer substantial gains or the possibility of substantial drops in value. They're considered high risk.

- Small-cap funds can provide notable rewards, but with the potential for severe losses. Again, it's a high-risk investment.

You may have noticed that there are no low-risk stock mutual funds. That, of course, is because there are no low-risk stocks. Stocks can always lose some of their value — or fail to grow — even highly respected stocks. And mutual funds will reflect those losses. Also, labels such as "large cap" or "growth" funds are frequently added by the fund manager and may be marketing tools. Take nothing for granted.

Risk haters are not without options when it comes to mutual funds. You can buy mutual funds with low to medium risk. That's because many mutual funds either don't invest in stocks at all or invest in stocks only partially. Mutual funds can also own debt instruments such as bonds. Obviously, with such funds you're not going to get the surging appreciation that a hot growth mutual fund can achieve — no 30 percent a year, or even close — but you'll have the peace of mind of knowing you'll be getting some growth with less chance of losses.

Here are some leading types of low-risk funds:

- Money market funds invest in certificates of deposit, U.S. treasury notes and other conservative investments. They keep your money out of danger and pay about what bank CDs pay. Risk is low.

- Tax-exempt money market funds invest in short-term municipal bonds. That means your money is very safe, and you don't have to pay federal taxes on the interest earned. Risk is low.

- Short-term bond funds can be either taxable or tax free. They have holdings in bonds from corporations or domestic and foreign governments, or both. Their risk level is fairly low.

- Long-term bond funds can be either taxable or tax free. They're a bit riskier than the funds listed above, but with higher potential income.

- Ginnie Mae funds invest in securities that represent government-backed home mortgages. They can offer a decent income, but they do entail some risk.

- Global bond funds invest in bonds from foreign companies and governments, as well as some U.S. companies and governments. They represent a moderate level of risk.

Real estate. Investing directly in real estate — that is, owning properties that produce income and, it is hoped, appreciate in value — tends to be as much a job as it is an investment. If you intend to create a new business and new responsibilities for yourself when you retire, then owning properties could be for you. It can be rewarding and profitable. But if you don't appreciate that your property and your tenants will require your attention — not to mention the ongoing expenditure of money for upkeep, taxes and insurance — then it's best that you don't get into it. It could be a real headache, and it's nothing like buying a stock, a mutual fund or a CD.

Even if you don't care to get up at 5 a.m. to plow out your apartment building's parking lot, you can get into real estate indirectly. A real estate investment trust (REIT) is bought and sold like a mutual fund. Three types are available — REITs that invest in property (such as office buildings or apartments), REITs that invest in mortgages or securities backed by mortgages, or hybrid REITs that do both.

Just as if you were buying a stock or a mutual fund, you need to do your homework when buying a REIT. The quality of management is important, as is the quality of the properties that the REIT has invested in. Look at the REIT's income from operations, which reflect the fund's earnings.

Although REITs are subject to dramatic fluctuations in the real estate market — booms and busts — they tend to provide good income and at least a bit of growth. Still, they entail much greater risk than bonds and shouldn't be considered as the bedrock of a retirement investment strategy.

Life insurance. There are two primary types of life insurance:

Term life is purely insurance against the possibility that you unexpectedly lose your life due to illness or accident. It provides your beneficiaries — whomever you choose — with a cash settlement of a predetermined amount. That predetermined amount, ideally, is what your survivors will need to get along comfortably without you. The rates go up as you get older (and possibly sicker) and face an ever greater risk of dying.

Whole life insurance, on the other hand, performs two functions at once: It will provide your beneficiaries with a predetermined death benefit in the event that you die. And it serves as a kind of tax-deferred savings account. That is, the part of the money you pay that is not devoted to paying the life insurance premiums will build cash value over the policy term. Whole life premiums begin at a higher level — because of the investment component — but remain predictable. When you withdraw money from the policy, you pay income taxes on the earnings.

However, the cash value that you're hoping for is not entirely predictable. The rosy rate of return that the insurance agent suggests at your sales presentation is just an estimate. Your return may vary significantly depending on how well the company's own investments perform, the number of policy cancellations and the mortality rate of policyholders, among other factors.

Some experts maintain that you'll do just as well or better buying term life and investing the difference. And you won't be tied into a single investment for many years, as you are when you buy a whole life policy. Whole life is only likely to pay off if you stick with it for the term of the policy. If you bail out early, you may lose those savings you thought you were tucking away.

One possible advantage of whole life is that it compels the reluctant saver, who never can seem to find money to put into that IRA or 401(k), to tuck away some money. When the insurance company presents you with the prospect of losing your balance if you don't pay its bills, you're more apt to write those checks.

Universal life insurance lies between term and whole life insurance. Universal life offers you the ability to buy the basic insurance policy at a low premium (like term life insurance) but then gives you the flexibility to increase your premium and put the additional money into a savings account within the policy. Often the policy is a variable universal life that offers several different investment options.

Annuities. Offered by life insurance companies, annuities let you put as many after-tax dollars into them as you care to, with all of their appreciation tax deferred. You can buy an annuity with a lump sum or make monthly payments. When you withdraw money from the annuity, you're taxed on the appreciation, not on the principal. If you happen to die, the life insurance company will pay your heirs the greater of either the amount you've put into the annuity or its current market value.

An annuity can either pay you regularly for the rest of your life, or for a certain period ending with a lump sum payment. If you make the former choice, be aware that if you die fairly soon after retirement, the insurance company may keep the part of the annuity you haven't taken.

You can buy two types of annuities. Variable annuities invest your money in stock or bond mutual funds. The yield varies according to how those funds do, though a minimum rate is generally promised. Fixed annuities pay you a specified rate only. You must be age $59\frac{1}{2}$ to begin taking money out of your annuity.

Whatever you choose in terms of buying annuities, remember that you're paying taxes both on the money you put into an annuity and on the income you're taking out of it after retirement. That's why you should maximize your tax deferred retirement investments before buying an annuity: The money you invest in an employer retirement plan, such as a 403(b) or a 401(k), is pretax dollars and is taxed at your ordinary income tax rate upon withdrawal. The money you invest in a Roth IRA (see page

121) is after-tax dollars, and the balance is tax free at the time of withdrawal. The money you invest in a traditional IRA could be pre-tax or after-tax dollars, depending on your income level at the time you invest the dollars. It's best to invest in employer retirement plans and IRA accounts before considering an annuity.

Pensions and retirement accounts

Classic pensions. The classic pension, or defined benefit plan, is made up of contributions made toward your retirement by your employer. The money doesn't come out of your salary. The size of your pension generally depends on your length of service and your final salary. The longer you're at the job, the bigger your pension gets. However, few of these pensions offer any protection against inflation.

These standard pensions are not portable. They may reach a certain size by the time you quit your job, but that's all you're entitled to when you retire. You start a new pension from scratch at your new job, if the new company offers one. If you plan to put much reliance on a classic pension when you reach retirement, it's best to stick to a job as long as possible. Job hoppers generally do not come out as well.

If you're an average earner at a typical company, you can probably rest assured that your pension will be there for you even if your company has problems in the future. Most pension plans are insured by the Pension Benefit Guaranty Corp., a federal agency that guarantees a certain maximum monthly payment for you, depending on when you retire and whether your plan covers beneficiaries. Government entities, religious and fraternal organizations, and some other types of businesses are not covered.

To find out more about the Pension Benefit Guaranty Corp., go to its Web site at *www.pbgc.gov*. The Administration on Aging offers pension counseling programs. You can find information at *www.aoa.dhhs.gov/factsheets/pension.html*.

Defined contribution plans: 401(k). If you work at a for-profit company, chances are you'll be able to set aside a percentage of your pretax salary in a defined contribution retirement plan — a 401(k).

And generally it's not only your money that goes into the plan — some employers match a portion of your contribution to the 401(k) plan.

You can invest a percentage of your pretax salary into your 401(k), up to a percentage specified as the legal limit (15 percent). Above that limit you can make after-tax contributions, if your employer permits. Including your pretax and after-tax contributions, and your employer's contributions, you can set aside up to 25 percent of your salary for retirement. Your pretax contributions are deducted automatically. The money that your employer invests in the plan can vary — from a small percentage of your pretax contribution up to 100 percent of it, or more. It's up to your employer to make that decision.

If you contribute to a 401(k), you'll be given certain investment choices. These might include a selection of stock mutual funds, money market funds, bond funds and your own company's individual stock. If you change your mind about where you want your dollars to be invested, you'll be able to make changes. But you may have to wait to make any changes until a date specified in the rules of your company's defined contribution plan.

If you leave your employer, you can leave the balance invested in your employer's plan or complete a direct rollover of the balance to your new employer's plan, or to a traditional IRA account. A direct rollover means the balance is payable directly to your new account, not to you. If the check is made payable to you, your previous company will be required to withhold income taxes on the balance. If you are under $59^1/_2$ the IRS could assess a 10 percent penalty for early withdrawal if you do not invest 100 percent of the balance in your new account.

Also keep in mind that if you haven't been fully vested — that is, been at work long enough to qualify for 100 percent of your employer's contributions — you won't get all of the money that your employer contributed.

Defined contribution plans: 403(b) and 457. If you work at a nonprofit organization or a government entity, you may be able to participate in a 403(b) or a 457. You will be given certain investment choices for both plans. Employers may contribute money to the plans, but it's not as likely as it would be with a for-profit employer. Once again, you're allowed a maximum contribution based on your salary.

Traditional IRA. If you receive compensation (earned income) and you're not age $70^{1}/_{2}$ or older during the tax year, you can contribute to a traditional individual retirement account (IRA). You're allowed to contribute up to $2,000 a year. This contribution may be in pretax or after-tax dollars, depending on your income level. You

Saving money by sharing housing

If you're an older homeowner who's finding it difficult to cover all your expenses with your retirement income, shared housing may offer a solution. Many people share housing for the companionship and security it offers. But if you own the home, the arrangement also can mean added income, in the form of rent. Before you go ahead and find someone to share your home with, you'll want to check local regulations to make sure you don't violate zoning ordinances. You'll also want to seek advice about how the additional income will affect your Social Security checks or whether your taxes or insurance will go up.

Finally, consider your personality. While the extra income might be welcome, keep in mind that you'll be opening your home to another person who will expect the rights and privileges of a tenant. Are you willing to give up your privacy and to make compromises? Can you accept sharing your kitchen and bathroom with someone else? How will you handle chores and other responsibilities? How compatible are you with your potential renter? In addition, you'll want to make sure that you have a sound method for qualifying any potential candidates and develop a strategy for what to do if the arrangement is not working out.

Advice about home sharing can be obtained from the National Resource and Policy Center on Housing and Long Term Care (*www.aoa.gov/Housing/SharedHousing.html*). The National Shared Housing Resource Center (*www.nationalsharedhousing.org*) offers a directory of programs on a state-by-state basis.

can put your IRA money into almost any sort of investment — an ordinary savings account, a CD, mutual funds, individual stocks or REITs. You can have as many IRAs as you want, but you're limited to the contribution of $2,000 a year.

SEP-IRA. If you're self-employed or own your own small business, you can put up to 15 percent of your pretax income — up to a specified maximum — into a simplified employee pension-IRA (SEP-IRA). This can be in addition to having an ordinary IRA.

Roth IRA. The Roth IRA is a newer kind of individual retirement account for the self-employed, small business owners and employees with certain income limits. Instead of receiving pretax dollars when you're paying into it, the Roth IRA receives dollars that have already been taxed. That is, you use your after-tax dollars, up to $2,000 a year. The benefit of the Roth IRA comes when you take the money out after retirement — you pay no tax at that time. With a traditional IRA, you do pay income taxes as money is withdrawn. The amount depends on your tax bracket at the time of withdrawal.

If it is used properly, the Roth IRA has several advantages over the traditional IRA. First, you're not obliged to withdraw any funds from it until you want to. A traditional IRA requires that you start drawing on it no later than April 1 of the year after the year during which you reach $70^{1}/_{2}$. With a Roth you could hold it in reserve — letting its contents grow for you or your heirs — until you're 70, 75 or beyond. Also, you can withdraw your principal whenever you want. After all, you've paid taxes on it already. Any interest your Roth has earned, however, is penalized 10 percent if you withdraw it before age $59^{1}/_{2}$.

If you're comfortable with a little more discomfort today and your income is below a certain level, the Roth IRA makes a lot of sense. However, if you can't afford to contribute $2,000 without the deduction, you probably should use a traditional IRA.

Earned income

For some retirees work remains a part of their lives. Some work out of necessity, because their income from Social Security and retirement investments isn't adequate to meet their needs. Some work because they enjoy the stimulation and challenges it provides, the contact it gives them with other people or the feeling that they're filling a need. Of course, it's nice to have some extra income, too.

Whatever your motivation for working after retirement, chances are that there'll be plenty of opportunities for you. Many employers are eager to find competent, responsible part-time employees. And retirees who've worked the better part of a lifetime know something about the work ethic. Retirement also represents a good opportunity to try a new line of endeavor — perhaps going back to school and picking up a new skill.

You may even be able to make some arrangement with your present employer to do a phased retirement. You decrease the amount you work, gradually taking less of a paycheck, but gaining more free time. Meanwhile, your pension remains unaffected.

Creating your financial plan

If you're the type of individual who makes meticulous plans, keeps close track of your income and expenses, sticks to a predetermined budget and generally avoids nasty financial surprises, you should have no trouble getting your finances ready for retirement. For you, creating a retirement plan and following it should be a piece of cake.

If you're not particularly good at planning and budgeting and keeping financial discipline, now would be a good time to try to change. Without these qualities, you could find yourself coming up unpleasantly short of funds as you launch into your retirement. You need to analyze the situation you're currently in, decide what it is you want to do with your retirement and make a plan to achieve those goals.

Everyone has different paths to achieving retirement goals. The retirement ambitions and resources of one person will not be like those of another. If you had children in your early twenties, your retirement will be radically different from someone who had children in their late thirties or early forties. If you're single, your path to retirement isn't the same as that of a married person.

Setting goals

To achieve the secure retirement you'd like to have, you must begin by setting a target date. Perhaps you crave an early retirement; perhaps you'd like to keep working well into your late 60s or early 70s. Whatever it is, regard that date as an approaching deadline whose requirements must be met in time. This is a long-term goal.

But don't forget short-term goals. Every year until retirement, you'll want to put money away. You'll want a similar plan to pay down your debt every year so that you enter retirement without much debt burden. Set and meet goals like these every year, and you should be in good shape for retirement. Some experts recommend saving at least 10 percent of your annual pretax income.

For both long- and short-term goals, make written plans, work hard to follow them and compare your actual results with what you've specified. But these goals shouldn't be carved in stone. Keep the flexibility to change them if your work or personal situation changes significantly.

Getting down to basics

Setting long- and short-term goals is a fine notion. But how do you attain them? Here are some general tips:

- Know where your money goes by keeping track of all significant expenditures, from the cost of your weekly groceries to your house mortgage.
- Know where your money is by keeping an inventory of all your cash accounts, investments, retirement accounts, real estate holdings, and so on. You can keep this information — which should be updated regularly — in a ledger book or in one of the popular personal finance software programs. If you use software, be sure to make backup copies frequently.
- Create a budget and try to follow it.
- Before all else, pay down as much high-interest, nondeductible debt as you can. If you're a long way from clearing out your debt, try to refinance at lower rates. For instance, transfer credit card balances to accounts with lower rates. If you feel that

you're in over your head, seek out a qualified credit counselor to help you create a debt reduction plan. Better yet, seek ways to elimnate all debt before you retire.

- Participate in your employer's retirement plan by contributing as many pretax dollars as you're allowed to. If possible, put money in any other tax-deferred plans that are available to you — as much as you can afford, to the legal maximum. A good minimum amount is 10 percent of your paycheck, whether your contributions are taxable or tax-deferred dollars.

- Start making the transition to retirement today by living on your anticipated retirement budget. Think of this as a reality test.

- Understand that taxes and inflation will have a negative effect on your retirement nest egg. What seems like a lot of money today may not be in the future. Plan accordingly. Keep in mind the Rule of 72 (see page 97) when assessing the effects of inflation: If annual inflation is at 8 percent, the purchasing power of a dollar will be reduced by one-half in 9 years ($72 \div 8 = 9$).

- Be smart when it comes to the equity you own in your home. Keep in mind that if you take out a home equity loan, you expose yourself to the risk of losing your home if you're unable to make payments. You also put your house at risk if you use it as collateral for a loan — whether yours or another family member's.

- As people get older, they become targets for fraud and scams. Their money is stolen by fraudulent telemarketers, contractors who do bad work or no work, bogus "bank examiners," "stock brokers" with hot tips, and so on. Never give your money to anyone who doesn't provide at least three solid references and can't wait for you to think it over. And remember that old bit of advice: If it sounds too good to be true, it almost certainly is.

- Don't forget that most basic step to achieving your retirement goals — stay healthy. If you use tobacco, do your best to stop. Put the money you'd spend on cigarettes into a money market account and watch it grow. If you don't exercise, get active. If you drink too much, cut down. If you don't visit a doctor regularly, consider starting. Leading a healthy lifestyle might make a big difference in how much of your retirement income goes toward health care expenses.

Selecting a financial planner

Should you be your own financial planner? Perhaps you've made enough income to meet your needs and have figured out how to avoid going too far into debt. Taking the money you've saved, you put it into mutual funds, treasury notes, stocks, bonds or other investments. You've learned from those experiences, maybe made a few mistakes, but your investments have grown, and you're comfortable with your plan. Some people enjoy financial planning and have the skills and interest required to be successful.

Others do not. Perhaps you don't have the knowledge, interest or time to handle your financial duties as effectively as possible. Maybe you've added a major new expense, such as a baby, or had an unexpected windfall. Maybe you just need help to clean up your financial act. In these cases a professional financial adviser can

---

Questions to ask a financial planner

The Certified Financial Planner Board of Standards *(www.cfp-board.org)* recommends that you ask the following questions when selecting a financial planner:

What experience do you have?

What are your qualifications?

What services do you offer?

What is your approach to financial planning?

Will you be the only person working with me?

How will I pay for your services?

How much do you typically charge? (Hourly, flat fee or percentage? By the hour or as a percentage of the assets under management?)

Could anyone besides me benefit from your recommendations?

Have you ever been publicly disciplined for any unlawful or unethical actions in your professional career?

Can I have it in writing?

help. This person will help assess your current financial status, suggest changes to optimize your returns, develop plans to meet your future goals and periodically review and update these plans.

Anyone you hire to provide you with financial planning help should be properly qualified. Look on a planner's business card for credentials such as certified financial planner (CFP) or chartered financial consultant (ChFC). Good planners may also be lawyers, certified public accountants or chartered life underwriters. Be skeptical of anyone who pushes certain investments or promises you amazing results in a short period. The adviser who promotes a slow and steady approach to wealth building is apt to be a reasonable choice. And be sure to ask for references — clients who've been with the adviser for 3 or more years.

Estate planning

Even though you've done a great job managing your retirement finances, it doesn't change the fact of your mortality. Some day you will die — it is hoped, at a ripe old age — and what remains of your estate will go to your spouse, your children and grandchildren, to some favorite charitable cause or perhaps to a variety of heirs. How smoothly and effectively your assets are transferred into their hands depends largely on how you arrange now for your estate to be disposed of. You want to know that the right people will benefit from your life of hard work and sound financial planning, and now's the time to see to it that they do.

Assessing your estate

Before you begin to make plans for your estate, you need to take an inventory of just what that entails. It includes everything you own that conceivably has some value. Major items in your estate may include:

- A home
- Additional real estate
- Ownership interest in a business
- Life insurance

- Investments
- Retirement accounts
- Savings accounts
- Vehicles
- Other personal property

Making a simple will

The simplest way to assure that your heirs get what you want them to have is to create a will. About half of all Americans, however, don't have wills in effect when they die. And then guess who gets to decide who gets what from your estate? A probate judge whom neither you nor your heirs have probably ever met. If you don't have heirs and die without a will, your state government can claim your money and property.

Accelerated death benefits

If you find yourself suffering from a terminal illness, you may have the option of drawing funds from a life insurance policy to pay for health care or other expenses during this difficult time — while you're still alive. This type of benefit is called an accelerated death benefit or living death benefit. It can take the form of a rider to a policy you already have or it can be a policy bought just for the purpose. To qualify for an accelerated death benefit, you must have certification from your physician that you're terminally ill with a year or less to live. Usually you get the face value of your policy less a discount.

An alternative way to get money out of your life insurance policy, in the event of a terminal illness, is called a viatical settlement. Arrangements are made for some other party — often a company or investor group — to buy your life insurance policy. You get a certain part of the policy's face value, generally 50 percent to 80 percent. And you remain the insured. But the policy's new owner — who continues to pay the premiums — becomes the beneficiary and receives the policy's proceeds upon your death.

An attorney can draft a will for you that describes your estate, gives the names of your beneficiaries and what they're to receive, makes any other special provisions if you wish, and names an executor (a manager for your estate).

Most wills go through probate court, to some degree or another. The smaller your estate, the simpler that process is apt to be. It rarely takes more than a year.

Living trusts

Another way for you to dispense your estate to your heirs is to create what's called a revocable living trust.

A living trust also is a legal document created by a lawyer. It describes how you want your estate distributed after you die and names a trustee to see to its execution. Its major benefit is that it allows your assets to be passed along to beneficiaries without going through the process of probate. You also have the option of specifying how your property should be handled in the event that you become incapacitated. It does not take effect until you transfer your property to the trust.

Minimizing taxes

If you're like most Americans, you want to assure that your heirs get as much of your estate as possible, and the government gets as little as possible by way of taxes. Several good options are available that will help you minimize or eliminate the money your estate owes to the federal government and the state you live in:

- To begin with, no federal estate taxes are owed on estates of $675,000 (for 2001) or less. By 2006 that figure rises to $1 million.

- Give money or property to your heirs during your life. You can give $10,000 a year tax free to anyone you choose. A couple can give $20,000 a year. This amount may increase, depending on inflation.

- You can pass any amount of money or property to your spouse while you're alive. However, this may increase the federal estate tax liability upon the death of the last surviving spouse.

When losing a spouse means losing financial security

For older women, widowhood or divorce often raises the specter of financial hardship. An added handicap for these women is that some of them don't have confidence in their own ability to understand and manage their personal finances. Their husbands may have taken care of all the financial chores, leaving them unexposed to the basics of maintaining budgets and handling investments. Worried about their financial futures, many are unable to make decisions or end up erring on the side of caution — and lose potential income as a result.

That's why it's important for each partner in a marriage to understand the overall financial picture and be a part of the planning process — even if he or she is not naturally inclined to do so. For widowed or divorced spouses, the best way to avoid a financially bleak future is to learn what you need to know today.

- A bypass trust (also known as a credit shelter trust) can provide a surviving spouse with income during his or her life from a deceased spouse's estate, while reducing or eliminating heirs' estate tax exposure after the death of that surviving spouse.

- A charitable remainder income trust (CRIT) is created when you give a valuable asset (such as a stock holding) to a charity. The charity in turn sells that asset and puts the funds into a trust that pays you income for the rest of your life. At your death the charity takes possession of the trust's assets.

- A charitable lead trust (CLT) does exactly the opposite of a CRIT. Instead of you receiving income from a trust created from your assets, the charity receives the income. At your death your heirs receive the assets of the trust.

Estate counseling

Whether your estate is simple and small or large and complex, it's important to enlist the aid of an experienced attorney, certified public accountant or other appropriate professional in charting out the disposition of the money and property you've spent a lifetime accumulating.

Estate laws can be complicated and difficult to understand, and without the help of a professional to guide you through them, you could be setting up your heirs for a larger tax liability than you ever thought possible.

Disclaimer: The content in this chapter is presented as general information and is not intended to be a comprehensive overview of all your financial options. Nor is it meant to imply an endorsement by Mayo Clinic of any type of financial plan, product or service. Investing your money is a complicated and serious process that is constantly affected by conditions in the marketplace and changes in tax law and government monetary policy. There is no guarantee that an investment product bought today will perform the same from year to year. Your best advice is to research your choices as thoroughly as possible and, when in doubt, to consult a trusted professional financial or investment adviser.

Your health care

- **Take nothing for granted when it comes to your health.**
- **Be cautious in selecting health care providers.**
- **Regular health checks are essential.**
- **Prepare an advance directive, and make it known to your loved ones.**

No matter how old you are, it's important to keep a close eye on your health and to catch problems early, when treatment is most successful. But the older you get, the more important this becomes. As you grow older, your body changes. The physical problems you encounter can be much different — and more wide-ranging — than in years past. Almost 9 out of 10 people age 65 and older have at least one chronic illness, such as arthritis, heart disease or diabetes. And nearly 1 in 3 people over 65 have at least three such illnesses.

As an older adult you're also more prone to drug reactions and adverse drug interactions because your body chemistry changes. Even nonprescription drugs that you used to take without any problem may now produce surprising side effects.

In addition, your symptoms — if they show up at all — can be hard to detect and can have greater consequences if left untreated. For instance, you could have a mild heart attack without realizing it. That's because you might experience little or none of the chest pain that would usually alert you to the problem.

Also, your road to recovery is often a much longer journey than in the past. That's partly because when you grow older you typically experience some decline in organ function, meaning your body might not work as efficiently as it used to in healing itself. You don't bounce back as quickly as you did in the past.

Still your senior years can be the greatest time of your life — a time when you may be free from the daily grind — able to spend more time with family and friends and in pursuing whatever else interests you. But to get the most out of these years and enjoy life to the fullest, you'll want to keep close tabs on your health. That starts by making sure you have the best doctor you can find — one suited to your unique needs.

What to look for in a doctor

If you don't already have a main doctor, often called a primary care doctor, now is the time to find one. This is the physician who helps you make most of your medical decisions and who oversees the care you get from specialists. If you wait until you're sick and in a rush for relief, you may be forced to turn over serious treatment decisions to a doctor you don't know and who doesn't know you. That kind of uncertainty can make matters worse. When you're sick is not the time to scan the Yellow Pages looking for a doctor.

You'll probably want to choose one of three kinds of doctors as your main doctor — a family practitioner, an internist or a geriatrician. A family practitioner provides health care for people of all ages. An internist treats adults, and may have had additional training in a specialty such as heart diseases. A geriatrician is trained in family practice or internal medicine, and has had additional training in caring for older adults.

To receive a medical license, all doctors have to graduate from an accredited medical school and go through at least one year of training afterward. That's the minimum. But for your care, you need a doctor specially trained and experienced in treating adults — one who has completed work beyond the minimum. This extra work is usually called a residency and involves 2 to 6 years of supervised training. This extra training makes a doctor eligible for certification by the board of a given medical specialty. Afterward, the doctor must pass the certifying exam. Family practitioners, internists and geriatricians have all gone through this extra training.

Before you start looking for a doctor, think about what you most want in a doctor. Make a list, identifying the essentials as well as other features that would be nice but aren't absolutely necessary.

At the top of your list, put these three essentials:

- Trust

- Ability to communicate

- Availability

You need to be able to trust your doctor's advice about your health care. You need a doctor who will take time to listen to your concerns and who will talk to you with words you can easily follow. You'll want a doctor who's not too rushed to explain the medical term for your diagnosis or to help you understand why you need certain tests. If you can't trust or understand your doctor, you'll probably not take the medical advice you get as seriously as you need to. And your health could suffer.

Make sure your doctor is easily accessible. Some insurance programs may try to assign you a doctor who practices in another town. Find a good doctor as close to home as possible. You'll be more willing to go see the doctor when you need to if his or her office is nearby.

As you work on your list, think about other doctors you've had. Consider what you liked and didn't like about them. Perhaps you liked the doctors who were friendly and emotionally involved in your care and didn't like the doctors who were strictly business and bossy.

If you're a woman, you may prefer a woman doctor. If you're a man, you may prefer a man doctor. If you have a chronic health problem, such as diabetes, you might want a doctor who has a subspecialty in that area.

Here are a few other questions to consider as you expand your list:

- Do you want a doctor practicing alone or in a group?

- How far away is the doctor's office from your home?
- Does the doctor accept Medicare or other insurance you have?
- Is the doctor allowed to admit patients to the hospital you prefer?
- Is the doctor part of a health maintenance organization (HMO)? If so, what restrictions does this imply?

How to find a doctor

Once you have an idea about what kind of doctor you want, identify several candidates. If you're on a managed care insurance plan, you may be limited to the doctors on the insurance company's list. If so, call the insurer to make sure you have the most current list.

Narrow your search

The best way to find a doctor is by word of mouth from trusted friends. So ask your friends, family, work colleagues and other trusted health care providers for recommendations. Be sure to ask what they like about the doctor, as well as any problems they've noticed. This can help you zero in on selected doctors.

Call the doctor's office

Once you've selected two or three doctors, call their offices. Tell the receptionist you're looking for a doctor and you'd like to speak with someone who could answer a few questions about the doctor and the office procedures. Take note of how the assistants respond to you because if you choose this doctor, you'll be working with these people. Are they courteous and helpful, or do they seem abrupt and inconvenienced by your call?

A good place to start is to find out if the doctor is accepting new patients. Next, ask if the doctor accepts your medical insurance plan.

Here are a few other questions you might consider asking:

- What's the doctor's special field of practice?
- Do you treat many older people?
- What are your office hours?

- How many days a week does the doctor see patients?
- Are evening or weekend appointments possible?
- If I call the office with a medical question, can I speak with the doctor?
- How does the doctor arrange to answer medical questions after hours?
- How far in advance do people have to make an appointment? (If longer than a month, the doctor is probably overloaded. You might want to look elsewhere.)
- How long do people generally have to wait in the office? (Expect a wait of less than 20 minutes.)
- How willing is the doctor to refer people to a specialist?
- How long will you be able to visit with the doctor? (Some HMOs restrict total time to less than 30 minutes.)

Verify credentials

Before you invest time and money in visiting a doctor, make a phone call or visit a Web site to confirm the doctor's credentials. If your doctor is board certified in a specialty, such as family practice, internal medicine or geriatrics, you can confirm this by checking with the American Board of Medical Specialties. You can call this organization at 866-275-2267 or log on to the Web site *www.abms.org*. The American Medical Association also has a Web site that identifies specialists. It's called AMA Physician Select, *www.ama-assn.org/aps/amahg.htm*.

To determine if any disciplinary action has been taken or may be pending against a doctor, call your state medical licensing board. For the number, look under state government listings in your phone book or call directory assistance. Keep in mind, however, that even the best doctors occasionally have legal problems. So don't let this be the only factor in your decision.

Visit the doctor's office

After deciding on your first choice of a doctor, make an appointment. You'll probably have to pay for the visit, even if all you want to do is get to know the doctor. With that in mind, you might as well schedule a checkup. Let the assistant doing the scheduling know that this is your first visit and that you'd like a little extra time to talk with the doctor.

If you're having an exam, follow the advice in the section "Getting ready for your checkup" on page 154.

As you did in your initial phone call to the doctor's office, when you arrive for your appointment pay attention to how the office staff treats you. Also make note of how long you have to wait. If it's longer than 20 minutes, ask about the reason for the delay. The office staff may have overlooked your name on the list. Or perhaps the doctor is delayed at the hospital, and you may choose to reschedule the appointment.

When you meet the doctor, feel free to ask about:

- His or her medical background
- Why he or she chose to practice in a certain field of medicine
- Whether he or she treats many people in your age group and with your particular medical problem (if you have any)

Trust your instincts

If you don't feel compatible with the doctor, try the next one on your list. You're more likely to follow the advice of a doctor with whom you feel comfortable. Doctors know it. So don't worry about offending them. Concentrate on your needs.

Specialists you may need

How do you know when you need a specialist or other health care provider, such as a physical therapist, a physician extender or a nurse practitioner? Generally, your main doctor will refer you to a specialist when you have a problem that warrants it. If you're concerned that you have medical problems not being adequately cared for by your main doctor, you might want to seek a specialist whose training and experience matches the problem.

Knowledge about diseases and treatment is growing so fast that specialties and subspecialties have emerged to help manage this information. A family doctor or internist, for example, can't possibly keep up on all the new findings in each area of health care from head to toe. Specialists are sometimes needed to perform many of the different diagnostic tests and to interpret the data. You and your main doctor will find it reassuring to have so many sources for specialized help with any complex health care problems that may lie ahead.

If you visit a specialist, ask that the records of your diagnosis and treatment be sent to your main doctor, who needs to keep track of your overall health care. Ask for a copy of the records for yourself. Also, next time you visit your main doctor, be sure to give a report of what the specialist did for you.

Specialists

Here's a brief list of specialists you might need as you grow older, along with the systems, diseases, conditions and therapies that they can help you with:

Allergist, immunologist. Allergies, such as hay fever and insect stings, as well as asthma and diseases of the immune system.

Audiologist. Hearing.

Cardiologist. Disorders of the heart, blood vessels and circulation.

Dermatologist. Skin diseases, which are common among older people and can be deadly.

Endocrinologist. Problems with the glands, which control your body's hormone system, including pituitary, thyroid, adrenals, ovaries and insulin-producing cells of the pancreas. You might see such a specialist for care of diabetes.

Gastroenterologist. Digestive diseases affecting the esophagus, stomach, colon, liver and pancreas.

Geriatrician. Aging and diseases of older adults.

Gynecologist. Female organs and diseases.

Hematologist. Diseases of the blood, including anemia, leukemia and lymphoma.

Nephrologist. Kidney problems.

Neurologist. Diseases of the nervous system, which includes the brain, spinal cord and nerves.

Orthopedist. Conditions affecting bones, joints, muscles, ligaments and tendons.

Oncologist. Cancer.

Physical medicine and rehabilitation specialist (physiatrist). Rehabilitation, especially through therapeutic exercises and techniques such as heat, cold, electrical stimulation and biofeedback.

Psychiatrist, psychologist. Mental disorders. A psychiatrist (a physician) can diagnose medical conditions and diseases and can prescribe drugs. A psychologist specializes in psychological assessment and counseling therapy.

Pulmonologist. Diseases related to breathing, such as asthma or emphysema, which primarily involve the lungs and bronchial tubes. You might also see such a specialist for sleeping disorders, such as sleep apnea and snoring.

Rheumatologist. Problems of the joints, muscles and connective tissues, which include arthritis. You might also see this specialist for immune conditions such as lupus.

Other health care providers

Nurse. If you're in the hospital, you'll probably see nurses more frequently than doctors because nurses provide most of the care. The nurses observe symptoms and listen to you describe them, help carry out the treatment plan and evaluate the results.

The initials *R.N.* after a nurse's name mean registered nurse. To be an R.N., a person must complete a bachelor's degree in nursing or a similar program, and then pass a licensing examination in the state where he or she plans to practice. Some registered nurses have postgraduate degrees.

The initials *L.P.N.* mean licensed practical nurse. The L.P.N. course of study is shorter, and the L.P.N. generally works under the supervision of an R.N.

Some nurses specialize. For instance, they might focus on pediatrics or cardiology. Some not only specialize but also become a nurse practitioner (N.P.). A nurse practitioner usually has at least a master's degree and performs many of the same basic tasks as a doctor — examining and treating people as well as writing prescriptions.

A nurse practitioner usually works in group practices, helping doctors manage the heavy load of office visits by diagnosing and treating people with the more common and less serious health problems.

Most N.P.s specialize in a particular area of health care, such as family medicine, adult health, pediatrics, neonatal care or geriatric care.

Occupational therapist. If you're injured or disabled, an occupational therapist helps you regain your ability to carry out everyday tasks, such as the activities required to make a living. The word *occupational* is misleading because the therapy isn't aimed solely at helping you get back to work, but at regaining the ability to do daily tasks wherever you are, at home or on the job: eating, dressing, bathing, homemaking and recreational skills. This therapist may recommend physical changes to your home or workplace — such as rearranging furniture or adding ramps and railings — to make it easier for you to get around and carry out your tasks.

Pharmacist. Your pharmacist is a good source of information about your medicine, whether it's prescription or nonprescription drugs. Since the pharmacist keeps a record of all prescriptions you buy at his or her pharmacy, it's helpful to use the same pharmacy for all your prescription drugs. This provides a double-check, to make sure you don't take a medication that reacts with something else you're taking. The pharmacist can also help you select nonprescription drugs that are best for you. But if you're taking prescription medicine, check with your main doctor before taking nonprescription drugs that are new to you.

Physical therapist. Like an occupational therapist, a physical therapist also helps injured and disabled people regain lost physical functions, using techniques such as exercise, massage and ultrasound. The focus here is to maximize physical ability and compensate for physical functions that have been lost.

Health care problems among older adults that may require physical therapy include:

- Arthritis
- Deconditioning
- Incontinence

- Joint replacements
- Osteoporosis
- Parkinson's disease
- Spinal cord injuries
- Stroke and other neurologic conditions

Physician assistant. Like a nurse practitioner, a physician assistant often helps relieve some of the patient care load of a doctor by diagnosing and treating people with some of the more common health care problems. Most P.A.s have at least a bachelor's

Questions to ask before surgery

Whether your regular doctor or a surgeon recommends surgery, you'll want to ask several questions:

What is done during the operation? Ask for a clear description of the operation. If necessary, perhaps you could ask the doctor to draw a picture to help explain exactly what the surgery involves.

Are there alternatives to surgery? Sometimes surgery is the only way to correct the problem. But one option might be watchful waiting, to see if the problem gets better or worse.

How will surgery help? A hip replacement, for example, may mean you'll be able to walk comfortably again. To what extent will the surgery help and how long will the benefits last? You'll want realistic expectations. If the surgery will help you for just a few years, before you'll need a second surgery, you'll want to know that up front.

What are the risks? All operations carry some risk. Weigh the benefits against the risks. Ask also about the side effects of the operation, such as the degree of pain you might expect and how long that pain will last.

What kind of experience have you had with this surgery? How many times has the doctor performed this surgery, and degree. They generally work under the supervision of a doctor, performing work assigned by the doctor. Working as part of the health care team, they take medical histories, treat minor injuries that may require stitches or casting, order and interpret lab tests and X-rays, and make diagnoses. In most states they can also write prescriptions.

In some clinics most of the routine care is given by P.A.s. You may not see the doctor unless you have a major problem.

Surgeon. Your primary doctor will help you find a good surgeon should you ever need an operation. If you need a joint

what percentage of the patients had successful results? To reduce your risks, you want a doctor who is thoroughly trained in the surgery and who has plenty of experience doing it.

Where will the surgery be done? Many surgeries today are done on an outpatient basis. You go to a hospital or a clinic for the surgery and return home the same day.

Will I be put to sleep for the surgery? Your surgery may require only local anesthesia, which means that just part of your body is numbed for a short time. General anesthesia puts you to sleep.

How long will recovery take? You'll want to know when most people are able to resume their normal activities, such as doing chores around the house and returning to work. You may think there would be no harm in lifting a sack of groceries after a week or two. But there might be. Follow your doctor's advice as carefully as possible. It comes from observing what has happened to other people who had the same surgery.

What will it cost me? Health insurance coverage varies. You may not have to pay anything. You might have a deductible to meet. Or perhaps you'll have to pay a percentage of the cost. The doctor's office can usually give you information about this, but also check with your insurance company.

Be certain to know if you are responsible for a flat co-pay — a set amount for the surgery — or if you have to pay a percentage of the bill. There is a big — and expensive — difference.

replacement, for example, you'll probably be recommended to an orthopedic surgeon, who specializes in operations involving joints, muscles and bones. When choosing a surgeon, try to select one who has performed a lot of the kind of surgery you'll be having.

Given the potential risks and costs of many surgeries, it often makes good sense to get a second opinion. Either you or your primary doctor can make the decision to get that second opinion. So don't feel you need to be secretive about visiting a second surgeon. Keep your main doctor informed.

Shopping for health insurance

The most expensive medical bills you'll ever have are probably yet to come. Are you ready? A surprising number of middle-class people are impoverished when they reach their 70s and 80s because they had too many holes in their health insurance safety net. Decide now how you want to fill those holes.

Medicare

Medicare is the federal health insurance program for everyone age 65 and older. You are eligible no matter how much money you have. To enroll, call the Social Security Administration at 800-772-1213. The TTY-TDD number for the hearing or speech impaired is 800-325-0778. It's best to enroll during the 7-month period that begins 3 months before the month of your 65th birthday and ends 3 months after the month of your 65th birthday.

Medicare has two parts — Part A and Part B. Part A pays for most of these services:

- Hospital stays
- Skilled nursing care in a nursing home for the first 20 days
- Some home health services for the first 14 days after a hospital stay

You do not pay premiums for Part A, but you do pay deductibles and co-pays.

Part B, which is optional, pays for most of these services:

- Doctor visits

- Outpatient hospital care

- Laboratory services

- Preventive immunizations and screenings

You pay a monthly premium for Part B. In 2001, the monthly premium is $50, deducted automatically from your Social Security check. In addition, you pay an annual deductible of $100. You also pay 20 percent of the amount Medicare approves for your medical bills. For example, if Medicare allows $100 for your doctor visit, you pay $20.

You may have heard the expression "accepting Medicare assignment." Doctors who accept assignment have agreed to charge you no more than what Medicare is willing to pay. You still pay the 20 percent co-pay and the $100 deductible, but you do not pay anything beyond that. Ask your doctor in advance if he or she accepts Medicare assignment. If not, your out-of-pocket expenses may be almost 10 percent higher.

Your choices. Medicare offers several types of health plans. No matter which you pick, you are still in the Medicare program.

Original Medicare. This is the traditional basic plan you are automatically enrolled in unless you choose another option. Most people stay with Original Medicare. It pays Medicare's share of your costs under Parts A and B. You pay the balance. You can use almost any doctor or hospital in the country. You receive all services Medicare covers, but no extra benefits.

Original Medicare with a supplemental policy. Strongly consider buying a supplemental policy if you have Original Medicare. They are called Medigap policies because they pay for gaps in coverage, that is, things that your Original Medicare does not pay for. A Medigap policy is a good way to fill some holes in your insurance safety net.

All private insurance companies that sell Medigap policies offer the same 10 levels of coverage. These are labeled Plan A through Plan J. Some levels pay only for Medicare deductibles and co-pays. More expensive levels pay for prescription drugs and home care.

Insurance companies must enroll you in the Medigap plan of your choice if you apply within 6 months of enrolling in Part B. This open enrollment period is offered only once. If you miss it, insurance companies in some states can refuse you Medigap coverage. Your Medigap insurer must renew your policy for life as long as you pay your premiums. You can switch to a different Medigap policy, but certain rules apply.

Medicare managed care. With Medicare managed care you receive care from a managed care plan. It might be a health maintenance organization (HMO), a provider-sponsored organization (PSO) or a preferred provider organization (PPO). All three are

If only

I had never heard of a living will. But after what happened when my husband died, I tell everyone I know, if you don't have one, get one.

Greg died at age 66 of chronic obstructive pulmonary disease. At first it made him short of breath and weak. Then his immune system weakened, and he got sick more often and took longer to get better. His heart had to work hard to get oxygen to his body, so it grew bigger to try to keep up. Eventually it couldn't keep up. After a series of heart attacks, his lungs filled with fluid, and he died of congestive heart failure.

It was a long and awful road to travel. After the heart attacks, they were always able to bring him back, but after each one, there was a little less of him there. Then he went into a coma.

The doctors asked if we wanted a "do not resuscitate" order on for him. That means if he were to have another heart attack, they would take no steps to get his heart started again. We had a family meeting in the intensive care unit waiting room. My younger son was against it. My oldest son thought it was best. I didn't know what to do. It was a nightmare.

The doctor asked if my husband ever completed a living will. I didn't even know what it was. He explained it's a piece of paper you fill out so family and doctors know what kind of medical care you want in case you can't speak your wishes.

He showed me a sample. It was easy to fill out, and it doesn't cost anything. Most hospitals and clinics have them. I read it over. What would Greg have written on this? Would he have wanted them to do everything medically possible even when there was no chance of him enjoying life again? I just didn't know.

variations on the same theme. A limited network of doctors and hospitals takes care of you, often at lower cost to you than if you were insured by Original Medicare. You don't need a separate Medigap policy if you join a Medicare managed care plan. That's because the managed care plan agrees to cover some of the same services Medigap plans do.

When you enroll in a managed care plan, Medicare pays the plan a fixed amount no matter how many services you need. That

Meanwhile, our family was torn apart in disagreement over what to do. The boys were at each other's throats, digging up old grudges and skeletons that had nothing to do with their father lying in a coma. There was just so much stress and bitterness and uncertainty. He's our dad, the youngest would say. We just can't let him die. Dad wouldn't want to live like this, the oldest would say. And there I was in the middle in an agony of indecision, staring at this piece of paper. Greg and I never even talked about this sort of thing. If only he'd filled out one of these papers.

The doctor said it was ultimately my decision. I hadn't slept and was functioning on pure emotion. I just couldn't sign the do-not-resuscitate orders. Greg had another heart attack. They resuscitated him. He stayed in a coma. A week went by. There was talk of moving him to a nursing home. Then he coded again. This time, they couldn't restart his heart.

By the time Greg died, the boys weren't speaking to each other. If Greg had signed a living will, it still would have been a terrible ordeal, but at least we would have known what he wanted. We had to guess, and this is not a guessing game. We all lost.

Widow — Sioux Falls, S.D.

Points to ponder

- Save your family grief and turmoil by discussing end-of-life wishes.
- Complete a living will and a power of attorney for health care, and let your family know that you've done so.
- Make sure your family knows where to find these documents.

means the health plan has a financial incentive to restrict services. You can only go to the doctors and hospitals that are part of that managed care plan. For that reason managed care plans may not be a good choice if you travel frequently or live in another part of the country for part of the year.

Managed care plans might save you money if you follow plan rules and only get the care your plan approves. You might also get extra benefits, such as prescription drug coverage and vision care. These plans offer the best benefits in states that receive higher Medicare reimbursements from the federal government — often but not always the more populated states.

Some managed care plans decide not to participate in the Medicare program. If your plan leaves Medicare, you will automatically be covered by Original Medicare until you find another managed care plan in your area. Or you can just stay with Original Medicare.

Private fee-for-service plans. In a private fee-for-service plan, you choose a private insurance plan that accepts Medicare beneficiaries. You can go to any doctor or hospital in the country. To enroll you must have Medicare Part A and Part B. You do not need a Medigap policy if you have this type of Medicare plan.

The insurance company, not Medicare, decides how much it will pay for services and how much you will pay. You get all the services covered in Medicare Parts A and B. You may also get benefits that Original Medicare does not offer. Your premiums and out-of-pocket costs may be higher than with Original Medicare. You still pay the Part B premium and usually an additional monthly premium. You will probably have a co-pay for each visit or service provided.

Medicare medical savings account. A Medicare medical savings account (MSA) is part insurance policy and part savings account. You buy one from a private insurance company. Medicare pays your MSA premium and deposits money in your MSA. You use the money in the savings account to pay for your health care.

Annual deductibles can be as high as several thousand dollars. You can pay that deductible out-of-pocket or with the savings account. You cannot buy a Medigap policy to pay the deductible.

Doctors and hospitals can charge you as much as they want above Medicare-approved amounts. At the end of the year, any money left in your MSA savings account stays there for future use.

You still pay the Part B premium. Some MSA plans let you go to any doctor or hospital. Others require you to stay within a preferred network. MSAs are so new that few companies offer them. To find out if anyone offers MSA plans in your area, call 800-Medicare. Ask for a free copy of *Your Guide to Medicare Medical Savings Accounts.*

Decisions, decisions. To research Medigap plans or other plan options, visit *www.medicare.gov.* This site has a telephone directory of plans available in your area. Local libraries and senior centers have information, too. Request an application form for plans that interest you and follow the instructions.

When choosing a Medicare plan that's right for you, consider these points:

Coverage away from home. If you travel often or live in another part of the country part of the year, make sure your plan covers you while you're away from home. Managed care plans offer only limited coverage while you're away.

Specialists when you want them. Medigap and fee-for-service plans let you see any specialist whenever you want to. Most managed care plans require you to see specialists who are part of the plan's network. Often you must get approval from your regular doctor first. Make sure the specialists you desire are part of your plan's network. If they aren't you'll pay much more out-of-pocket when you see them.

Limited budget. If you cannot afford unexpected health care costs, Original Medicare with a Medigap policy is probably the right choice for you. Certain managed care plans also might be a good choice for you because their costs are usually fixed.

Prescription drugs. If you have trouble paying for prescription drugs, consider a managed care plan. They usually provide equal or better drug coverage at less cost than do Medigap plans.

Employer retiree coverage. If you have good insurance through a former employer, Original Medicare is probably all you need. Do not give up good retiree coverage. It probably offers you more than Original Medicare combined with a Medigap policy. Many employers stop your retiree coverage as soon as you enroll in Original Medicare.

Medicaid

Medicaid helps people with low incomes pay medical bills. It also pays for nursing homes and other long-term care. To qualify for Medicaid you and your spouse must have a low income and very few assets. Each state has different rules. To find out if you qualify in your state, call your state department of social or human services. To find the office nearest you, look in the phone book or visit the Web site of the Health Care Financing Administration, the federal agency that administers Medicare and Medicaid, at *www.hcfa.gov*.

Most states let you choose any doctor or hospital in your area that participates in Medicaid. An increasing number of Medicaid recipients are enrolled in managed care plans, such as HMOs. Doctors and hospitals that participate in Medicaid must accept what Medicaid pays as payment in full. However, some states require you to pay small deductibles and co-pays.

Dual eligibility. Some people are eligible for both Medicaid and Medicare. For these "dual eligibles," Medicaid acts like a Medigap policy. That's because Medicaid pays for more services than Original Medicare does. The lower your income and assets are, the more Medicaid helps pay for your Medicare out-of-pocket expenses.

If you have a Medigap policy, but a change in your financial status makes you eligible for Medicaid, you can suspend your Medigap policy if you do so within 90 days of becoming eligible for Medicaid. If your financial status changes again and you lose Medicaid coverage within the next two years, your Medigap coverage will automatically be returned to you without penalty.

Medicaid and long-term care. Medicaid pays for more than half of all nursing home costs today and almost 70 percent of the care of nursing home residents. It also pays for at-home care.

The annual cost of living in a nursing home can exceed $40,000. Many middle-class couples get caught off guard. They spend their savings and assets paying for long-term care until they're impoverished and qualify for Medicaid. Some people deliberately spend down their assets or transfer wealth to other family members in order to qualify for Medicaid. Stricter laws now make this harder to do.

Medicaid is government welfare. If you use it to pay for long-term care, you may not get to choose the type of care you receive or the location where you receive it. If this concerns you, plan ahead and find a different way to pay for long-term care.

Long-term care insurance

Chances are you will need some type of long-term care in your life-time. How will you pay for it? Medicare and Medigap policies do not pay for most types of long-term care. Long-term-care insurance (LTCI) fills a big hole in your insurance safety net. It is one way to pay for long-term-care services you may someday need. These include:

- Nursing home care
- Assisted living
- Elder day services
- Home care
- Respite care

LTCI is expensive and not the right choice for everyone, but long-term care is even more expensive. An average nursing home stay costs $56,000 a year. Assisted-living facilities cost on average $26,000 a year. Elder day services charge $30 to $130 a day. Home care can cost an average of $12,000 a year.

Once you reach age 65, you face a 50 percent lifetime chance of needing a nursing home for some period of time. Half of us who reach 85 will need some type of long-term care. Not planning a way to pay for that care is why many older adults become poor.

Do you really need it? Most people buy LTCI for these reasons:

- Protect assets you plan to leave to heirs.
- Prevent the need for your family to take care of you or pay your bills.

- Help you stay independent in your home longer.
- Avoid having the government pay your long-term-care bills.
- Ensure you have more choice about where and how you receive long-term care.

LTCI buys you peace of mind. It is probably not the right choice for you if your income is low and you have few assets. Nor do you need it if you've saved enough to pay for long-term care, though you might still want to buy it to protect your assets.

Can you afford it? Do not buy LTCI if you cannot afford the premiums. As a general rule of thumb, do not use more than 7 percent of your annual income to pay for premiums. In 1999, the median annual income for buyers of individual LTCI policies was $42,500.

You can probably afford a good policy if:

- Your household assets are worth at least $75,000 a person, not including your house and cars
- Your household retirement income is at least $35,000 a person
- Paying the premium does not force you to change your lifestyle
- You can afford premium increases of 20 percent to 30 percent during the policy's lifetime.

Annual cost of the same 4-year policy at different ages*

Age at time of purchase	Average Annual Premium
50	$ 888
65	$1,850
75	$5,880

* Policy provides coverage of $100 a day for nursing home care, $50 a day for home care, a 29-day elimination period (deductible), 4 years of coverage, and 5 percent inflation protection. Remember that the costs will be much higher in 15 years.

Source: Health Insurance Association of America

At what age should you buy? The younger you are when you buy a policy, the lower your premiums will be. There's a trade-off, however. If you buy LTCI too young, you may pay many years of unnecessary premiums. You might not use your policy until you are in your late 70s. Decide when to buy based on your health, family medical history and finances. People between the ages of 55 and 64 buy one-third of all individual LTCI policies. Many experts agree that a good time for many people to buy is when they are in their 60s.

Your premiums stay the same once you lock in at a certain age. But, they can be increased if they are increased for an entire group of policyholders.

How much and how long? As a general rule, you should buy enough coverage to pay for at least two-thirds to three-fourths of the daily nursing home costs in your area. Most people buy policies that pay for 2 to 6 years. You may use the benefits all at once or on and off as needed. Policies that pay for 3 to 4 years are adequate for most people. The average nursing home stay is 2 1/2 years. Forty-five percent of nursing home stays last 3 months or less. About one-third last 1 year or longer. Twenty percent last 5 years or longer.

What to look for. It's impossible to know what kind of long-term care you may need. It's a good idea to buy a policy that covers at-home care as well as care in a nursing home. Decide if you want a policy that pays for home modifications, such as ramps and railings, that help you stay in your home as long as possible.

Virtually all policies now cover Alzheimer's disease and no longer require a stay in the hospital before benefits are paid. Most policies are guaranteed renewable. That means it cannot be canceled as long as you pay your premiums on time and you tell the truth about your health on the application.

Maximum daily benefit. The maximum daily benefit is how many dollars a day a policy pays for nursing home care. How much daily benefit you should buy depends on how much you can afford or want to pay out-of-pocket. It's generally a good idea to buy a daily benefit that pays for at least half to all of nursing home costs. Policies usually pay home care benefits at about half the nursing home daily benefit. For example, a policy that pays $150 a day for a nursing home might pay $75 a day for home care.

Duration of benefit. Deciding the duration of benefit that you want in your LTCI policy can be confusing. A 4-year policy does not mean that you only get benefits for 4 years. It means you get benefits until 4 years' worth of the maximum daily benefit has been used.

Pooled benefit policies. Pooled benefit policies provide a total dollar amount that you can use to pay for any type of long-term care, not just nursing homes. They are popular because they offer flexibility. They are more expensive than policies that pay fixed amounts for each type of long-term care.

Inflation protection. You'll pay more for a policy with inflation protection, but it's usually worth it. The costs of long-term-care services are rising about 5 percent a year. It could be many years before you use your policy. Inflation protection automatically increases your benefit amounts so they keep pace with rising costs.

One-time deductible. Choose a policy that requires you to satisfy the deductible only once during the life of your policy.

One-time elimination period. Choose a one-time elimination period. An elimination period is the number of days you agree to pay for your care out-of-pocket before the policy starts paying. For example, if you choose a 60-day elimination period and need nursing home care at $100 a day, you must pay $6,000. Shorter elimination periods cost more. Avoid policies that require you to meet the elimination period each time you need care.

Premium waiver. If you have a premium waiver in your policy, you are not required to pay premiums once you enter a nursing home or are receiving home care. You start paying premiums again when you are no longer receiving these services. Waivers are usually a good idea.

Tax-qualified vs. non-tax-qualified policies. Part of the premiums you pay for tax-qualified policies may be deductible on your federal income tax returns. But few people qualify for the deduction. To qualify you must itemize your deductions, and you must have medical expenses for the year that exceeded 7.5 percent of your adjusted gross income. You may deduct only a small portion of your premiums. The older you are, the more you can deduct.

Benefit triggers. Benefit triggers are requirements that you must meet before the policy pays for services.

- Pre-existing conditions. Policies often require a period of time to pass before they pay for care related to a health problem you had when you became insured.

- Activities of daily living (ADLs). These include things like bathing, eating, dressing and using the bathroom. Many policies start to pay when you can no longer perform two ADLs. It's a good idea to make sure bathing is included as one of the trigger ADLs because that's often the first activity people need help with.

- If you buy a policy that pays for home care, decide if you want to have benefits trigger once you need people to come to your house to cook and clean.

- Look for a policy that allows your doctor to decide when you are eligible to receive benefits.

- Choose a policy that lets you qualify for benefits because you either need help with activities of daily living or you have a mental impairment, but not both.

How to lower premiums. Consider buying a LTCI policy only for the female member of your household. Most nursing home residents are women. Half of all women 65 and older will spend some time in a nursing home. Men are more often able to rely on family for care.

If both you and your spouse want a policy, check for married couple discounts. You may also qualify for a discount if you are in above average health. Check to see if your employer or former employer offers LTCI, which usually means a group rate with lower premiums.

You can significantly lower premiums by not having inflation protection. In most cases this is not a good way to save on premiums. Instead, consider choosing a longer elimination period (the time before the policy starts to pay).

Nonforfeiture riders are an expensive extra you can probably do without. The rider ensures that if you stop paying premiums, you still receive part of the policy's benefits. Instead, be sure you can afford the premiums for the life of the policy.

Bargain-basement policies, especially from a company you've never heard of, might be a money-saving temptation. Don't buy one. If a policy doesn't cover what you need, you've wasted your money.

Ask the pros. LTCI is complicated. Simply deciding if you need it requires a good deal of thought and analysis. There are no easy, off-the-shelf answers. If you do buy it, scrutinize the fine print for restrictions and provisions. Most states require insurance companies to give you a 30-day free look, which means that after you sign the policy, you can return it within 30 days and receive a full refund.

It's a good idea to talk to an expert before you buy. Financial planners and attorneys who specialize in elder law can help you decide if you need a policy. They can also help you understand the fine print.

All states offer free health insurance counseling. Call the Eldercare Locator Service at 800-677-1116, which offers a free directory of aging services in every state.

For more information on Medicare, Medicaid and LTCI, visit these Web sites: American Association of Retired Persons (*www.aarp.org*), United Seniors Health Council (*www.unitedseniors-health.org*), Health Insurance Association of America (*www.hiaa.org*), American Health Care Association (*www.ahca.org*), and Health Care Financing Administration (*www.hcfa.gov*).

Getting ready for your checkup

You need periodic health examinations for two main reasons. First, the exam allows your doctor to identify medical problems early, sometimes before you develop symptoms. That's generally when treatment is most successful. Second, the preventive care you get at a checkup reduces your risk of developing certain diseases. For example, a blood test can tell if your cholesterol levels are turning a corner toward the unhealthy. And that can alert you to change your eating and exercise habits to ward off potential problems with heart disease or a stroke.

But have you ever wondered how often you should have a routine medical exam? Whether you need a checkup every year depends on your risk factors for specific diseases. If you're healthy, a general timetable for routine checkups is this:

- Twice in your 20s
- Three times in your 30s
- Four times in your 40s
- Five times in your 50s
- Annually after 60

If you'll need more frequent exams, your doctor will tell you how frequent.

In these exams expect your doctor to carefully review your medical history, including all of the prescription and nonprescription medicines you're taking. You'll receive a thorough physical examination, requiring you to disrobe. So wear clothes you can easily remove and put back on. You'll also be given screening tests to check for potential or emerging problems.

Keep up-to-date records

Knowing your own and your family's medical history helps your doctor more effectively diagnose and treat your problems — and anticipate potential problems on the horizon. But much of this information has to come from you. How can you keep track of it all?

Create your personal health planner. Here's some of the information to include:

Allergies. List any substances that you're allergic or sensitive to. These could include medications, food, pollen (note the season it affects you), mold, dust, insect stings, adhesive tape, latex, dyes used for X-rays. Also note whether you've had complications from anesthesia.

An ounce of prevention

They say fellows my age are supposed to get a physical exam every year. So I do. Every year, my doctor checks my prostate — not pleasant, but it's over and done with quickly. Lately, he's been giving me a prostate specific antigen (PSA) test, too. It's nothing fancy. They already take some blood to check for sugar and cholesterol. This PSA is one more blood test they do.

For 10 years, I aced the PSA test, scoring a 2, which is normal. Spring of '98, my PSA level shot up to 4. Three months later, I scored a 6.2. Time for a biopsy, the doc said. The biopsy showed I had prostate cancer.

Today, after undergoing radioactive seed implant treatment, I'm cancer free. My doc says I'm a classic case. My rectal exam was normal and I had no symptoms. If it wasn't for the PSA test, no one would have known I had cancer. And now I may be cured. The PSA was a pretty good investment.

62-year-old — Kansas City, Missouri

Points to ponder

- Everyone over age 60 should have a physical exam once a year. Schedule one every 2 years once you reach age 50.
- Preventive screenings when combined with a physical exam can detect problems not otherwise detectable.
- If you're a man over 50, ask your doctor about PSA testing.

Personal medical history. Record any illness or treatment that required hospitalization, surgery or emergency care. One by one, list the condition, treatment, hospital where the treatment took place, city and date.

Family medical history. Genes that run in your family may increase your risk of getting certain diseases. If your doctor knows who in your family had what diseases, you may reduce your risk of developing the same problems. "Family" means blood relatives, including brothers and sisters, father and mother, and grandparents. Information about aunts and uncles could be helpful, too, if you have access to it.

Record each family member's name and beside it note your relationship to that person, his or her health conditions, his or her age if alive, his or her age at death and the cause of death.

Personal immunization record. Keep a personal immunization record. Note the year you had each of the following illnesses or the most recent year you were vaccinated: tetanus, diphtheria, hepatitis A, hepatitis B and flu. For details about when and why you need these immunizations, see page 172.

Personal medication record. Tell your doctor about all the medicine you take. Include prescription and nonprescription drugs, vitamins, minerals and other supplements. Various drugs can cause problems when taken together. If you're an older adult, you're more susceptible to these problems because of your changing body chemistry and the increased number of medicines you may need.

At the very least, tell your doctor the name of each drug you take, along with the dose, how often you take it and what time of the day you take it. Be certain to mention over-the-counter medications and herbal preparations. To make sure there aren't mistakes in identifying which drugs you're taking, consider bringing them in their original containers so that your doctor can see them. The doctor may see a problem, for example, in a pharmacy's decision to substitute a cheaper generic drug for a name brand.

Make a list of questions

Before the exam think about what you want to discuss. Prepare a brief list of your main concerns, and put them in order of importance. At the top of the list, put one or two problems you worry about the most. For example, "My brother just had a heart attack, and I've been feeling some tightness in my chest. Do I have heart disease?"

Then identify less worrisome concerns. Perhaps you have to get up and use the bathroom several times a night, and it keeps you from getting a good rest. Or maybe your hands are stiff and sore in the morning. Don't overlook emotional problems. Make a note to ask your doctor about any continuing depression, nervousness or stress you've been experiencing.

Prepare to take equal responsibility for the success of your visit. Expect to ask all your questions and expect to be heard. Don't be a victim of a too-busy doctor. But remember, too, that the doctor's time may be limited. That's why it's important to focus on issues that matter the most.

Janet Vittone, M.D., a Mayo Clinic geriatrician, prepared the following list of potential questions:

- What are my risks of heart disease? Heart disease, including heart attacks and congestive heart failure, is the most common cause of death for both men and women over age 50.

- What are my chances of developing cancer? This is the second most common cause of death among older adults. For men, the most common cause of cancer deaths involves the lungs, the prostate or the colon. For women, it's the lungs, the breasts or the colon.

- What are my risks of a stroke? This is the No. 3 killer among older adults. You increase your risks if you smoke, have high blood pressure or have unhealthy levels of cholesterol (fat in the blood).

- Am I likely to develop diabetes? One in 10 patients over age 65 will develop diabetes.

- Do I need to be on all the medications I'm taking? On average a person over age 65 is on seven prescription medications. If you have concerns about the cost or side effects of these drugs, let your doctor know.

When the doctor orders tests

- How is the test done?
- What are the risks?
- What will it cost me?

After a diagnosis

- What's the long-term outlook for this condition? What happens to most patients?

- Do you have anything I can read about it?

- What can I do to improve my health?

- Are there classes I can attend or support groups I can join?

If your doctor prescribes a medicine

- How soon will the medicine begin to work?

- What are the possible side effects?

- How long will I have to take the medicine?

- Can I substitute a generic brand?

Signs and symptoms you don't want to ignore

Before your medical exam, think about any unusual symptoms you've been experiencing lately. If you're like many people, you may be tempted not to bother mentioning them. But some symptoms are early warning signs of medical problems you don't want to ignore. Treating the problem early can eliminate it or decrease the severity of complications later.

It's important that you describe your symptoms clearly and concisely. The more accurate your description, the better. A physical exam and tests are helpful in diagnosing a problem, but it's often your symptoms that first point the doctor in the right direction.

This checklist may help you describe your symptoms. Your doctor will know how to sort through your concerns. Expect the doctor to let you speak without being interrupted.

- What's your main problem?

- How long have you had it?

- How often does it occur?

- Do symptoms come and go, or are they persistent?

- What brings it on (activity, food, position, stress)?

- What time of day is it the worst?

- What makes it better (medication, stopping an activity)?

- What makes it worse?
- Is it associated with any other symptoms?

Here's a brief review of symptoms that might indicate serious problems. If you experience any of these, put them at the top of the list to discuss with your doctor. And if you don't already have an appointment for an exam, make one.

Blood in your stool. Often, blood in your stool is just a minor problem caused by hemorrhoids. The hemorrhoids tear, producing bright red blood that shows up in your stool, on the toilet paper or in the toilet bowl water. Sometimes the blood is darker in color, producing tarry black or mahogany-colored stools. Black stools mean the blood has been digested, and that you're bleeding from somewhere in your digestive tract — usually in the stomach or upper intestine. This could be an indication of an ulcer or cancer.

Vomiting blood. This is usually the result of injury or disease of the throat, the esophagus, the stomach or the beginning of the upper intestine (duodenum). The most common causes are:

- Ulcers
- A tear in the lining of the esophagus
- Inflamed tissue in your esophagus, stomach or small intestine
- Cancer of the esophagus or stomach

The blood is usually bright red. Occasionally, it appears black or dark brown and resembles coffee grounds, which indicates it has been partly digested either in your stomach or upper intestine. This often indicates a serious problem.

Coughing up blood. Coughing up blood usually indicates a problem in your lungs or windpipe. The blood is often bright red, frothy and salty. Possible causes:

- A bronchial or lung infection
- A blood clot in the lungs
- A blunt injury to the chest
- Lung cancer

Chest pain. Indigestion can cause chest pain. But so can a heart attack. The pain of a heart attack varies from person to person, but typically you'll feel a powerful squeezing pain in the center of your chest. It may last more than a few minutes, or it could go away and come back. In addition, you may experience intense perspiration.

Your chest pain may extend beyond your chest to your left shoulder and arm, back, and even to your teeth and jaw. Often the pain is caused by a blood clot blocking the flow of blood through one of the main arteries supplying your heart. This reduces or entirely cuts off the supply of oxygen to that part of the heart. As a result the heart muscle in the affected region dies.

Most often the clot that causes the heart attack forms in a coronary artery, narrowed by fatty deposits from the blood.

Skin problems. Your skin changes as you grow older. Generally, your skin gets thinner and loses some of its elasticity. After age 55 you may also pick up skin markings. Most of these are harmless, such as the common liver spots. A few types of marks can become cancerous, but the treatment is usually fairly simple.

See your doctor if a mole or another skin marking changes in color or size or if itching, bleeding or inflammation develops. Moles that are irregularly shaped, congenital (present from birth), mixed blue-black in color, or located around nails or the genitals need to be monitored carefully for such changes.

Dizziness or passing out. Reduced blood flow from your heart to your brain is the main cause of repeated dizzy spells. This can happen simply from getting up too quickly. Other, more serious causes include irregular heart rhythm, severe narrowing of the aortic valve in your heart or accumulation of fatty deposits in your neck arteries.

Other problems causing dizziness include changes in hormone levels, neurological disorders and side effects from drugs.

Confusion. Like dizziness, sudden confusion can be caused by restricted blood flow to the brain. Confusion, accompanied by trouble speaking or understanding, is a classic early warning sign of a stroke. Confusion can also be caused by drug side effects, low blood sugar levels, inadequate fluids in your body and nutritional deficiencies (especially niacin, thiamin, vitamin C or vitamin B-12).

Unexplained weight loss. Everyone's weight tends to fluctuate from day to day. But a sudden, unintentional loss of more than 5 percent of your weight within a few weeks — or 10 percent within 6 months — is uncommon, and reason for concern. Possible causes include:

- Difficulty swallowing, which leads to you eating less
- A digestive disorder that keeps your food nutrients from being adequately absorbed
- Pancreas or liver disease
- Cancer
- Depression
- Dementia

Tingling sensation or numbness. An ongoing problem with a tingling sensation or numbness can indicate that you have diabetes. Normally, your body breaks down part of your food into sugar that your blood transfers to muscles and tissue throughout your body, for energy and growth. But when you have diabetes, too much of this sugar stays in your blood. Over time high levels of sugar lingering in your bloodstream damage your nerves, which are nourished by your blood.

Nerve damage can produce a number of symptoms, but the most common are tingling and a loss of sensation in your hands and feet. Nerve damage happens slowly, over long months and years of high blood sugar. You may not even realize that you have nerve damage because you don't feel anything unusual. When your nerves are damaged, you can injure yourself and not even realize it. For example, you may burn yourself and not feel any pain. The injury, left untended, can develop an infection that may lead to more serious problems.

Tingling in the soles of your feet could indicate that you have a disk problem, such as a pinched nerve in your spinal cord. If you let that go, you can end up with permanent nerve damage.

Vision loss. A wide range of problems can cause vision loss. Sudden difficulty seeing out of one or both eyes can be a warning sign of a stroke. Strokes may occur near the optic nerve. But strokes in other parts of the brain that process the signal from your eye can also affect your vision, often causing problems with depth perception, general dimness of vision, or the loss of half a visual field.

Glaucoma is a vision problem caused by an increase in the pressure of the fluid (aqueous humor) inside the eyeball. With time this increased pressure damages the optic nerve, which carries visual impulses to the brain, so that vision is impaired. Unfortunately, the loss of vision is so gradual (often beginning with your peripheral vision) that many people permanently lose significant vision before the diagnosis is made and treatment is started. Only a small percentage of people with glaucoma have pain associated with it.

The incidence of glaucoma increases with age. Therefore, periodic eye examinations that include a check of vision and of pressure in the eyeball need to be done at 2- to 4-year intervals between ages 40 to 65 and every 1 to 2 years after that.

A detached retina is another serious vision problem that becomes increasingly likely as you grow older. In the back of the eyeball, behind the lens of your eye, is a jellylike substance called the vitreous. It's attached to the retina, the part of your eye that captures visual images. With aging, the vitreous tends to liquefy and cause the floaters that appear as specks or hairs in the field of vision. In vitreous collapse, the back portion of the vitreous may sag inward and pull on the retina. This can lead to retinal detachment, a serious threat to vision.

This complication is associated with a sudden increase in floaters and the appearance of flashes of light even when your eyes are closed or you're in the dark. If these symptoms suddenly appear, it is important to seek prompt consultation with an ophthalmologist. A retinal tear or detachment requires treatment to preserve vision.

One of the most common eye diseases among older adults is cataracts, which can cloud and distort the lenses in your eyes. About half of Americans ages 65 to 75 have cataracts to varying degrees. Fortunately, surgery to remove them is one of the most successful procedures done today.

Shortness of breath. When you experience shortness of breath, your lungs aren't able to get enough oxygen. Possible causes:

- Cornary artery disease, which reduces the flow of blood.

- Deconditioning, caused by a general lack of physical activity.

- Pneumonia, an infection or inflammation of the lungs. Such an infection can be caused by bacteria or viruses, or by inhaling dust, chemical irritants or food. Each year pneumonia kills more than 40,000 Americans, most of whom are over 65 years old.

- Bronchitis, an inflammation of the airways in your lungs, is usually caused by viruses, tobacco smoke, dust or molds and, sometimes, bacteria.
- Congestive heart failure, which causes fluid to build up in the lungs and feet.
- Lung cancer, especially if you cough up blood in the mucus.
- Sudden and severe shortness of breath can be caused by a blood clot that has moved from your leg to your lung, a condition called a pulmonary embolism.

At the checkup

During your checkup expect your doctor to carefully review your current symptoms, lifestyle and health habits, and medical and family history. He or she also will give you a head-to-toe physical exam. During this exam expect your doctor to:

- Check your height, weight, blood pressure and heart rate
- Check inside your mouth and throat
- Examine your eyes, ears, nose and skin (full body check for skin cancer every 2 to 3 years, annually after age 50)
- Feel for swollen lymph nodes in your neck, armpits and groin
- Listen for abnormal sounds from your heart, lungs or abdomen
- Feel for abnormalities in your abdomen, especially your liver, spleen or kidneys
- Feel and listen to pulses in your neck, groin and feet (checking for adequate circulation)
- Tap your knees to check reflexes
- Do a breast and pelvic exam (for women)
- Examine testicles for lumps or swelling (for men)
- Insert a finger into your rectum — called a digital rectal exam — to check the size of your prostate gland (for men)

Screening tests

Regular screening tests are the best way to catch potential problems in the early stages when odds for successful treatment are greatest. Which screening tests are right for you? Only you and your doctor can make that decision. However, we've compiled a list of 15 tests generally recommended for healthy older adults. If you're at risk of developing a particular disease, your doctor may order additional tests.

Cholesterol. Cholesterol is a waxy type of fat in your blood. Too much of it can clog your arteries, which can raise your blood pressure, make your heart work harder and put you at risk of heart attack and stroke. For every 1 percent you lower your total cholesterol, you cut your risk of heart attacks, strokes and other cardiovascular problems by 2 percent.

A cholesterol test is actually several blood tests. It measures your total cholesterol as well as low-density lipoprotein (LDL or "bad") cholesterol, high-density lipoprotein (HDL or "good") cholesterol and triglycerides, another chemical form of fat. Bad cholesterol deposits fatty residue on your artery walls, while good cholesterol carries it away from your arteries and to your liver for disposal.

The test is done by taking a blood sample after an overnight fast. You'll want to have the test every 3 to 5 years if your cholesterol levels are within normal ranges. Desirable ranges vary depending on your age, gender and health, so you'll need to talk to your doctor about what levels are appropriate for you. But here's a general review of the levels.

Understanding your cholesterol test

Blood fat	Recommended	Borderline	High risk
Total cholesterol	Below 200	200–239	Above 240
LDL	Below 130	130–159	Above 160
HDL	Above 45	35–45	Below 35
Triglycerides	Below 200	200–400	Above 400

Blood pressure. Blood pressure is determined by the amount of blood your heart pumps and the resistance to blood flow in your arteries. Narrowed arteries, such as those clogged with fatty deposits, limit the blood flow. The narrower your arteries, the harder your heart must work to pump the blood. Also, the longer high blood pressure goes untreated, the higher your risk of heart attack, stroke, heart failure and kidney damage.

To get your blood pressure measurement, an inflatable cuff is wrapped around your upper arm. It measures the amount of pressure your heart generates when pumping blood out through your arteries (systolic pressure) and the amount of pressure in the arteries when your heart is at rest between beats (diastolic pressure).

Have your blood pressure taken whenever you see your doctor, or at least every 2 years. You're at increased risk of high blood pressure if you're 35 years of age or older, overweight, inactive, have a family history of high blood pressure or are black.

Here's a chart to help you interpret your blood pressure measurement.

Understanding your blood pressure reading

	Excellent	Normal	High normal	High
Systolic (the first number)	120 or less	Less than 130	130–139	140 or above
Diastolic (the second number)	80 or less	Less than 85	85–89	90 or above

Colon cancer screening. Several tests are commonly used to detect colon cancer, along with growths (polyps) on the inside wall of your colon that may become cancerous. Many people skip colon cancer screening because they fear embarrassment and discomfort. But the test could save your life. Not only can it detect cancer early, when treatment is most successful, it can detect the precancerous polyps that doctors can easily remove, preventing cancer from occurring.

Get the screening every 3 to 5 years after age 50. You may need it sooner and more often if you're at increased risk of polyps or cancer because of your family history or because you have inflammatory bowel disease.

The exam methods are:

- Digital rectal exam
- Fecal occult blood test
- Flexible sigmoidoscopy
- Colonoscopy
- Colon X-ray (barium enema)

In a digital exam, the doctor uses a gloved finger to check the first few inches of your rectum. More thorough methods are generally used in addition to this simple exam.

The fecal blood test checks for blood in your stool. It can be done at your doctor's office or at home. However, not all cancers bleed, and those that do often bleed intermittently. Intense research is under way to determine if a more accurate stool test can be developed, such as diagnosing cancer cells in the stool (fecal colonocite). There's also research into whether taking aspirin or other nonsteroidal anti-inflammatory drugs can reduce colorectal cancer risk.

In the flexible sigmoidoscopy (sig-moi-DOS-kuh-pee), a doctor examines the lower part of your colon — which is where most colon cancer starts. This exam is done by inserting a flexible fiberoptic tube, called an endoscope, into your rectum. The procedure can be done in a few minutes. Polyps can be painlessly removed during the procedure. When polyps and early-stage cancers are found and removed before they've produced any symptoms, the cure rate is nearly 100 percent. That's why this kind of screening is so important.

A colonoscopy (ko-lon-OS-kuh-pee) is much like a flexible sigmoidoscopy, but more extensive. The difference is that the scope is longer and the doctor can examine your entire colon. The procedure

Feeling strong now

I avoided doctors because if there was bad news, I didn't want to hear it. Besides, I knew the lecture I'd get, but I didn't have time to exercise and eat right. I was 53 — an overweight, out-of-shape successful trial attorney who just couldn't stay away from the cigarettes. It took a three-vessel bypass to wise me up.

When the brakes get applied to your life as suddenly as they did to mine, you do a little thinking. Sylvia and I would retire in another 10 to 15 years and then who knows how long we'd have. Not long for me, I thought, unless I clean up my act.

I talked to some friends, did a little research and found a doctor I liked. Why did I like him? He wasn't some white-coated know-it-all. He gave me choices, instead of orders. He listened. We were partners. What I liked most was his sense of humor. "Look," he said. "Are you sure you want to quit smoking? The medical profession counts on guys like you. You're good for business." I got the picture.

Point made. Challenge accepted. I got on the program — weight training, rowing machine, lots of walks with Sylvia. I cut back on the cigarettes. That's right, I didn't quit. Eventually I did, but it's not easy. I started eating heart-healthy, which meant less saturated fat and more beans and rice and such. I make a mean black beans and rice casserole, by the way.

I feel great. I'm 32 pounds lighter. My blood pressure's down and so is my cholesterol. I don't huff and puff after mowing half the yard. My body just feels tighter and stronger. My golf game's improved, I think because I've got a bigger and stronger swing. I'm convinced exercise helps me think more clearly, too. Sylvia may be stuck with me longer than she thought.

Trial attorney — Minneapolis, Minn.

Points to ponder

- Exercise is the closest we come to a fountain of youth.
- It's never too late to undo the damage.
- A fit older person is healthier than an unfit younger person.
- If you don't want to collect your pension, don't bother with regular exercise.

takes about half an hour, and is currently the most effective screening method in use. An alternative to colonscopy is sigmoidoscopy combined with a colon X-ray.

An experimental screening technique is showing promise. It's called a virtual colonoscopy. It allows the inside of your colon to be examined using computer-generated images taken from outside your body. Also called CT (computerized tomography) colonography, this procedure involves a quick, 2-minute CT scan — basically, a highly sensitive X-ray — of your abdomen. Computer imaging then creates a multidimensional view of your colon. Before the scan your intestine is cleared of any stool so that air can be used to inflate the colon. Researchers are looking into whether the scan can be done without the usual bowel preparation.

Fasting blood sugar. A fasting blood sugar test checks for diabetes. It measures the amount of sugar in your blood. The test involves taking a blood sample after an overnight fast. Get the test if you're 45 or older. If your results are normal, repeat the test every 3 to 5 years. It you're at high risk of diabetes, get tested younger and more often. Your risk increases as you grow older, if you are overweight, have a family history of diabetes or are from one of the following racial groups: American Indian, black, Hispanic.

Mammogram. A mammogram is a breast X-ray to detect cancer and precancerous changes. Your breasts are gently compressed between plastic plates while a radiology technologist takes X-rays of your breast tissue.

Your risk of cancer increases with age and is higher than normal if you have a family history of breast cancer or had prior abnormal breast biopsies.

You need a mammogram every year after you turn 50. Before age 50 the recommended frequency depends on your risk factors, so ask your doctor for advice.

Pap test. A Pap test checks for cancer and precancerous changes in the cervix, the opening at the bottom of the uterus. Your doctor inserts a plastic or metal speculum into your vagina. Then using a soft brush, the doctor gently scrapes a few cells from your cervix. The procedure generally takes only a few seconds. The doctor then puts the cells on a glass slide and sends it to a laboratory for microscopic examination.

Get your first Pap test at age 18 or at the beginning of sexual activity. Additional Pap tests need to follow every 1 to 3 years. After three consecutive annual Pap tests with normal results, you and your doctor may decide on less frequent testing. For women who've had a hysterectomy for a noncancerous condition, routine Pap tests aren't necessary because the uterus is gone.

You're at increased risk of cervical cancer if you've had a sexually transmitted disease, multiple sex partners, history of cervical, vaginal or vulvar cancer, or are a smoker.

Prostate. As mentioned above, the digital rectal exam is used to check the size of the prostate gland. Another prostate test is a blood test to measure the level of prostate-specific antigen (PSA), a protein produced by the prostate gland. A high PSA level can indicate prostate cancer and noncancerous conditions. If you are a man over age 50, ask your doctor about PSA testing.

Blood chemistries. A blood chemistries test provides information about how well your organs, such as your liver and kidneys, are working. The test does this by measuring levels of substances in your blood, such as sodium, potassium, calcium, phosphorus and blood sugar, as well as liver enzymes, such as bilirubin and creatinine.

Blood cell count. A blood cell count, also called a CBC (complete blood count), helps detect the presence of many health problems, including anemia, infections and leukemia. The test measures:

- Hemoglobin (reveals the oxygen-carrying capacity of your blood)

- Hematocrit (percentage of blood volume made up of red blood cells)

- White blood cells (ward off infection)

- Platelets (enable your blood to clot, for healing of wounds)

Blood amino acid. Too much homocysteine (ho-mo-SIS-teen), an amino acid in your blood, can damage your arteries and put you at higher risk of heart problems and a stroke.

B complex vitamins — B-6, B-12 and folic acid — help reduce levels of homocysteine. As you age, your body becomes less efficient at absorbing B vitamins. This means you need to make sure you get enough of the vitamins.

There are no formal recommendations about when your homocysteine levels should be tested. Some doctors advise testing people in families with a history of narrowed arteries (atherosclerosis) and those who have cardiovascular disease.

Urinalysis. A urine specimen allows the lab to search for substances not normally found in urine. The presence of sugar points to diabetes. White blood cells may indicate an infection. Red blood cells can signal a tumor or a problem with the kidneys, ureter or bladder. Bile suggests liver disease.

Electrocardiogram. An electrocardiogram is a test in which electrodes are attached to your body to measure the pattern of electrical impulses from your heart. This test helps identify injury to the heart muscle, irregular rhythms, enlargement of a heart chamber or damage caused by a heart attack. Get a baseline test by age 40, and repeat the test as recommended by your doctor.

Your risk of heart problems increases as you grow older. You are also at increased risk if you have high blood pressure, high cholesterol, or a family history of heart problems, or if you are overweight or inactive.

Hearing. During a hearing test the doctor checks your speech and sound recognition at various volume levels to screen for hearing loss. You're at increased risk of hearing loss if you have been exposed to loud noises (such as gunshots and heavy machinery), had frequent ear infections or are over the age of 60.

Get a baseline test by age 60 or earlier if you suspect hearing loss.

Bone density. A bone density test is a quick, painless X-ray scan of your lower back and hip region to detect the loss of bone mass. A loss of bone mass can increase your risk of fractures (a condition called osteoporosis).

Get a baseline test by age 65 or earlier if you're at higher than normal risk of developing the condition. Your risk increases if you had early menopause, aren't taking hormone replacement therapy after menopause, have a family history of the condition, have taken cortisone medication for extended periods or are a smoker.

Immunizations

Nobody likes to get a shot. But immunizations protect you against diseases that would be far more unpleasant.

Here are the main immunizations you need to keep up-to-date. If you've lost track of when you had your shots, you can have a blood test to measure your immunity to these illnesses, which will tell whether you've had the diseases or immunizations. The following are general recommendations. Your doctor may add other immunizations based on factors such as your health, travel plans and job.

Flu (influenza). The flu is a viral infection spread from person to person by breathing infected droplets from the air. Get a flu shot every year if you're 50 or older. Others at high risk and who need a shot annually are those with chronic diseases (such as asthma or emphysema), those on immune suppressing medications and those such as school teachers, nurses and doctors, who have contact with a lot of people.

Pneumonia. Pneumonia is an infection, often from bacteria, that attacks your lungs and can spread to your bloodstream. It's common, serious and can be fatal, especially in older adults. If you're 65 or older, get immunized. Get the shot when you're younger if you have a chronic medical condition, such as heart disease or asthma, that increases your risk of infection. One shot lasts a lifetime for most people. But a booster shot more than 6 years after your first shot is advisable if you're at high risk or if you were immunized before age 65.

The shot helps protect you from bacterial (pneumococcal) pneumonia, but not pneumonia from other sources, such as viruses, fungi and other microbes.

Hepatitis A. Hepatitis A is a viral infection of the liver transmitted primarily through contaminated food or water. Immunization requires two shots with at least 6 months between shots. People at highest risk include those with liver disease or blood-clotting disorders, along with those traveling to areas where clean water and modern sewage disposal aren't available.

Hepatitis B. Hepatitis B is another viral infection of the liver, but it's often transmitted through contaminated blood. Immunization requires three shots during a 6-month period. You're at high risk if your work puts you in contact with human blood or body fluids, if you're on dialysis, if you've had multiple sex partners or if you've received donated blood products.

Tetanus. Tetanus is a bacterial infection that develops in deep wounds, such as a puncture from a rusty nail. Get a shot every 10 years. If you suffer a deep and dirty wound and your last booster shot was more than 5 years earlier, get a new booster within 48 hours after the injury.

Diphtheria. Diphtheria is a bacterial throat infection spread by breathing infected droplets from the air. The immunization schedule is the same as for tetanus, and both are generally given in the same shot.

Taking your medicine

If you're like most Americans, your medicine cabinet is a miniature warehouse of medication: tablets, capsules, lozenges, syrups, suppositories, creams, powders. As you grow older, you'll probably find the cabinet getting fuller and the range of medication getting broader. One-fourth of all prescription drugs in this country are used by people over age 65.

You can get the latest information about many specific medications by consulting our Mayo Clinic Web site at *www.MayoClinic.com*. Three topics, however, are especially important for older adults taking medicine.

Drugs that don't mix
As your medication needs increase and you find yourself taking several kinds of medicine each day, the danger of harmful drug interaction increases as well. Your main doctor may prescribe certain medicine. A specialist may prescribe others. You may add non-prescription medicine that you buy at the store.

Unfortunately, the action of one drug can be changed by the action of another — either blocking the desired effect or magnifying it to dangerous levels. Even seemingly harmless, nonprescription drugs can react this way when mixed with common prescription drugs.

You are at increased risk not only because older adults tend to take more medicine but also because of the changes in your body. As you grow older, lean muscle tissue decreases and fat increases. Many drugs are designed to be stored in fat tissue. And since you have more fat, the drugs can accumulate to higher levels. Also, your liver and kidneys become less efficient at breaking down and eliminating drugs — so the medicine stays in your body longer, with potentially dangerous side effects.

Keep your main doctor up-to-date on all the medicine you're taking. Sometimes doctors prescribe new drugs without reviewing what you're currently taking. Stay alert to that, and ask if the new drug will react to anything else you're taking.

If you're taking several drugs, it's all too easy for you to get confused and occasionally take too little or too much of some medicine. But as you grow older, the mistakes can grow more dangerous. Develop a method of making sure you take the right medicine at the right time. For example, set up a routine so that you take the medicine at the same time and the same place. Pillboxes and medicine calendars can help you stay on track. Select a pharmacy that's near your home and use it for all your medicine needs. Get acquainted with one pharmacist and talk to him or her frequently.

Brand name vs. cheaper generic

Many medications are available under the brand name of the company that first developed them and also as cheaper generic brands. The company that creates a drug gets exclusive rights to sell it for several years, to recoup development costs. When the patent rights expire, other drug companies can make and sell the drug. And they usually do so at much cheaper prices.

Though generic drugs are less expensive, some doctors say certain ones aren't made to the same standards as the original brand-name drugs. The filler that makes up the bulk of a tablet, for example, might be different than the original. And this can affect the potency of the drug it contains.

You and your physician need to determine whether you should use brand-name medicine or a generic equivalent.

Nonprescription drugs

Over-the-counter drugs, as they are sometimes called, are those you can get at your local pharmacy without a prescription. These include aspirin, cold remedies, pills for aches and pains such as menstrual discomfort, and creams for rashes. Some medicine can react with other drugs you're taking. And because of changes in your body as you age, certain drugs will affect you differently than they did when you were younger. Decongestants, for example, can make you so confused that people may wonder if Alzheimer's disease is setting in.

Among the wide variety of nonprescription drugs available are herbal, vitamin and mineral supplements not subject to strict control by the Food and Drug Administration (FDA). By an act of Congress in 1994, the FDA was relieved of its power to require drug companies to conduct expensive testing to prove the strength and safety of products labeled dietary supplements. By passing this law, in response to a grassroots letter-writing campaign, Congress acknowledged that consumers wanted the freedom to decide for themselves if herbs and supplements would help them.

Clinical studies have proven some supplements safe and effective. And research has weeded out several dangerous herbs. But the effectiveness and safety of many others still hasn't been established. Whether you're taking herbs, vitamins or other nonprescription medicine, your primary doctor needs to know about them.

Alternative treatment

Sometimes conventional medical therapy can't cure your problem, or it produces major side effects. For these reasons some people seek what doctors call alternative or complementary therapies. Many doctors in our country are reluctant to endorse these

Does the fountain of youth flow from a needle?

Inside you may feel 25, but your body keeps reminding you that you're not. You tire easily. Your knees hurt. And the only part of you that's thinning is your hair. You wonder about those anti-aging products you've seen advertised. Can they really make Father Time do an about-face?

One experimental anti-aging therapy that's getting more popular involves the synthetically produced human growth hormone (HGH). Your pituitary gland produces HGH, which builds muscle and bone and is responsible for growth spurts in children. The hormone tapers off after adolescence.

For the past 35 years, doctors have been prescribing HGH injections for children who are unusually short (due to a pituitary gland disorder) and for adults whose bodies produce so little of the hormone that they suffer from premature aging and other physical problems.

Although it is not standard practice, some doctors are now using HGH for the off-label purpose of helping people fight the natural aging process. Some high-profile HGH users, including celebrities, claim the hormone burns fat and reduces body weight, builds muscle and bone density, sharpens vision, softens skin, thickens hair, enhances memory and renews energy and sexual vitality.

The hormone is expensive. Available only by prescription, the injections can cost more than $1,000 a month and are not usually covered by insurance.

Besides being expensive, HGH has possible side effects: fluid retention, joint pain, diabetes, high blood pressure, carpal tunnel syndrome and breast development in men.

Some studies do suggest HGH has anti-aging benefits, but these studies have been small. And most doctors say it's too early to draw solid conclusions from them. The National Institute on Aging warns there's no proof HGH can prevent aging, but there is proof it has health risks. Until more studies are done, the best approach is caution.

approaches because they don't know enough about them to make a judgment. Nonetheless, a growing body of evidence indicates that certain alternative medical practices could have a role in treating some diseases.

Several therapies are used especially among older people.

Acupuncture. Acupuncture, a 2,500-year-old Chinese medical practice, involves inserting thin needles under your skin. Researchers say this stimulates your body's release of painkilling chemicals. To find a physician who has acupuncture training, call the American Academy of Medical Acupuncture at 323-937-5514.

Joint manipulation. Some chiropractors and osteopaths use joint manipulation to relieve the symptoms of osteoarthritis, claiming it relaxes the tissue around the joints and improves circulation. It's unclear whether this works.

Copper bracelets. For decades some people have advocated wearing copper bracelets to fight arthritis pain. They theorize that traces of copper pass through your skin and neutralize free radicals, which are toxic molecules that damage cells.

Wearing copper jewelry is probably harmless — its only known side effect is discolored skin. Most doctors find little evidence to recommend copper jewelry as a therapy for arthritis because scientific research supporting its effectiveness is scarce.

Other common alternative approaches. Other common alternative medicine approaches include aromatherapy, bee venom, gold rings, herbal treatments, magnets, snake venom and nutritional supplements. Before trying any alternative therapy, research it. Ask your doctor for information. Check the library, or consult a reliable Web site (such as *www.MayoClinic.com* or *www.nccam.nih.gov*).

Planning ahead

It's never easy to think about your death or getting so sick that you can't communicate. Nevertheless, it's in the best interest of you and your loved ones to prepare for both possibilities by creating an advance directive. The term *advance directive* refers to legal instruments that are used to make your wishes known regarding the extent of medical treatment efforts you want used on you if you become unable to communicate. They include a living will and a durable power of attorney for health care.

Put everything in writing. Each state has its own laws regarding advance directives. To view or download state-specific forms, contact the national organization Partnership for Caring at 800-989-9455 or visit its Web site *www.choices.org*. Once the forms are completed, give copies to your doctor, your surrogate decision maker and, perhaps, other family members. It's important to make sure your advance directives are accessible and used when needed.

Living will

A living will tells your doctor how you want to be treated when you're no longer able to communicate. You can direct your doctor to use, not use or stop treatment that helps keep you alive when you're terminally ill — such as paddles to shock your heart, treatments involving a breathing machine and tube feeding. Your living will should also mention views on organ donation.

Most states require doctors to honor these wishes. And even in those few states that don't, most doctors understand their duty to honor the requests of the people they are caring for, no matter how those requests are expressed.

Medical advances and your views about medical care are subject to change. So once you've created a living will, review and update it periodically, and communicate any changes to those involved.

Durable power of attorney for health care

In addition to a living will, you may consider entrusting a relative or a close friend with the power to make medical decisions for you when you're not able to make them for yourself. A living will is usually limited to life-prolonging treatment, but a durable power of attorney for health care covers situations not anticipated in your living will. A person with a power of attorney can make decisions on a broad range of health care issues, such as speaking on your behalf if you suffer an incapacitating stroke, dementia or an irreversible coma.

If you want to authorize someone with power of attorney, choose someone you trust and are comfortable with. He or she should understand fully your medical care philosophy and wishes. It also may be helpful, but not necessary, if this person lives close to you. Talk with the person you choose about what kinds of treatment you would want or not want in specific situations. Give copies of your power of attorney and living will to your loved ones and to your main doctor.

Even if you decide against a formal power of attorney, at least speak with your family and friends about how you would prefer your health care to be handled. By choosing someone now, you avoid the possibility of having a stranger appointed to this role by the court.

Who should prepare advance directives?

Any competent adult age 18 or older may prepare an advance directive. Those under age 18 may prepare a declaration but, by law (in most circumstances), parents or the health care provider is not required to honor it.

You're not required to prepare an advance directive. You do not need an advance directive in order to receive health care. However, if you feel strongly about what you would want done under certain medical circumstances or who should call those shots for you, an advance directive is a good idea.

Medical personnel will follow your advance directive to the fullest extent possible, consistent with a reasonable medical practice standard. That standard refers to the responsibility your physician has in determining what, if any, treatment is appropriate.

Consider organ donation

Each day about 60 people in this country receive an organ transplant. But another 16 people on the waiting list die because not enough people donate organs. Currently, about 60,000 wait for life-saving organs. Unfortunately, only about 6,000 organs are retrieved after donors' deaths each year. Hundreds of thousands more people are waiting for a life-enhancing transplant, such as those to restore sight or replace burned skin.

You can donate organs: heart, kidneys, pancreas, lungs, liver and intestines. And you can donate tissue: cornea, skin, bone marrow, heart valves, bones and connective tissue.

There's no age limit. Newborns and older adults have been donors. The deciding factor is the health of the organ or tissue, not the donor's age. Donation will not disfigure your body or interfere with an open casket funeral.

To become a donor, indicate your intent on your driver's license, in your living will or by carrying a donor card. Be sure to tell your family, since a family member is often required to sign a consent form. For a donor card, contact the following government Web site: *www.organdonor.gov.*

By becoming a donor, perhaps the pain your loved ones feel at your loss will be eased by knowing that in your last act, you helped others in great need.

Consider an autopsy

An autopsy is a detailed examination of a body to determine the cause of death. Fifty years ago about half the people who died in hospitals had autopsies. Much of what doctors know about diseases has been discovered or confirmed through autopsies. Unfortunately, fewer than 10 percent of the people who die in hospitals today have autopsies. The family often considers an autopsy degrading. Yet the procedure, which usually takes 1 to 3 hours, doesn't affect open casket funeral plans.

There are several reasons to consider requesting an autopsy.

Hereditary disorders. During an autopsy, the doctor may find something that can alert your family members to genetic problems they may have inherited and can protect themselves against.

Emotional comfort. Some family members may have felt as though they could have done something to prevent your death. In the case of a fatal heart attack, they might berate themselves for not insisting that you take it easier. But an autopsy might reveal a heart disease that could have taken your life at any time.

Insurance settlements. Knowing the cause of death can help resolve disputes that will affect the insurance benefits your family receives.

Helping medical science. The medical community learns from autopsies. The connection between smoking and lung cancer, for example, was confirmed by autopsies. The information helps evaluate treatment therapies and provides statistical data that influences government spending for health care. An autopsy is a way for you, in death, to help the living.

Funeral plans

The cost of a traditional funeral and burial can run $10,000 or more (cremation costs less). That makes it one of the most expensive purchases older adults face.

For this reason more and more Americans are either setting aside money to cover the expenses, or they're entering into contracts with funeral homes and prepaying for funeral packages. Nearly one out of three Americans over age 50 have prepaid some or all of their funeral expenses.

Either approach is a good idea because it takes tremendous pressure off your loved ones when the last thing they need is a $10,000 worry.

If you decide to buy a funeral package — whether it's just a cemetery lot or an entire package that also includes the casket, vault and services — it's a good idea to shop around. There's nothing wrong with selecting a funeral home or a cemetery based on location and reputation. But if you check at only one place, you may pay too much. Call or visit at least two funeral homes and cemeteries. The Federal Trade Commission's "Funeral Rule" requires that funeral homes — though not cemeteries — disclose prices by telephone. Many will mail you their price lists.

If you're buying a package, be sure to get prices for the casket, the outer burial container (often required by cemeteries to prevent the ground from sinking) as well as the funeral home's general services:

- Initial consultation
- Copies of death certificates, since you may need more than a dozen to settle matters such as insurance claims, social security issues and pension benefits

- Transportation of the body to the funeral home then to the burial site

- Preparing the body for burial

- Use of the facilities for visitation or a memorial ceremony

- Other options, such as flowers, music or preparing obituary notices

It's hard to think about such things while you're still healthy. It's even harder to set aside the necessary money. But if you do, your loved ones will know you did it for them.

Chapter 7

Roles and relationships

Take-home messages

- Don't try to go it alone.
- Circumstances change. Be adaptable.
- Know how to help others.

From your first breath on earth until your very last, you will be continually involved in relationships. You are born to parents and probably live with siblings, who bind you to your family of origin. You acquire childhood friends, then perhaps a spouse. Maybe you have children of your own and create a new family with its own dynamics, idiosyncrasies and traditions.

Good relationships nourish you in every stage of life. In them, you find comfort in times of trouble, encouragement when things get difficult and joy in shared experiences. You have fun together, but you also know that loyal relationships come with willing shoulders both of you can cry on. If you're smart and lucky, you'll accumulate alliances that will give you — and allow you to give — comfort, while shrugging off the ones that don't. These relationships are your safety net.

As you age, secure connections become even more crucial. Studies show that if you have just a few relationships or only poor ones, your risk of death will be two to four times greater than that of those who've surrounded themselves with many people they care about and who care about them — regardless of age, race and personal habits. In fact, having a dependable group of friends and family is one of the most reliable predictors of longevity.

There's no denying the solace that comes from good relationships. As the American novelist Pearl S. Buck wrote, "The person who tries to live alone will not succeed as a human being. His heart withers if it does not answer another heart. His mind shrinks away if he hears only the echoes of his own thoughts and finds no other inspiration."

But a life filled with people who care has its practical aspects, too. Consider how a social network of family and friends can benefit you, especially as you get older:

- Friends and family make it easier for you to give and receive affection, which strengthens your immune system and may keep you healthier.

- You're more likely to seek prompt medical attention when you have loving friends and family to remind you to go to the doctor or to take you there themselves.

- You're more apt to engage in healthful behaviors when you surround yourself with a like-minded social network that might, for example, launch an exercise program or give up smoking together.

- You can get help with practical matters, from financial questions, to trimming a tree, to choosing the right doctor.

- You can improve certain mental tasks by using your mind on everything from playing games to conversation.

In this chapter, we'll look at how maintaining good relationships can be one of the best ways to live a long and healthy life. We'll also discuss how roles and relationships change over time: how you may take care of aging loved ones in your middle years, then move on to being taken care of yourself. We'll also look at the role of caregivers, what it means to be one and how that's changing, too.

Getting connected

Families used to be closely connected. Grandparents lived near their grandchildren and were there to provide countless opportunities for learning and discovery, to say nothing of baby-sitting relief for the middle generation. Sometimes they moved in with their kids, creating three-generation households under one roof. Although such living conditions may cause their own tensions, studies have shown that living with extended family increases longevity.

In fact, the lack of social relationships may be a major health risk, putting you on par with someone who has high blood pressure, smokes or doesn't exercise. Fifty percent of Americans don't even live in the same state in which they were born. And generations rarely share a home now. In 1960, for example, 40 percent of people over 65 lived with an adult child. By 1999, the number had dropped to 4 percent. Siblings scatter in all directions, marrying and establishing families far from each other. Instead of supporting their relatives in practical, everyday ways, 21st-century Americans often rely on child care, neighbors and business associates.

As for friends, most people don't stay in one place very long. Childhood pals either get left behind or move out in their own widely diverse directions. In fact, the U.S. Census Bureau reports that the average person moves 11 times in a lifetime — and many will relocate much more often than that.

If this describes your situation, you can't wait until the children are grown or a spouse dies or you hit retirement to seek out your support system. Your support system inevitably will shrink as you age. That's why it's important to keep it current as you go through life, adding new friends as others depart. "If a man does not make new acquaintances as he advances through life, he will soon find himself left alone," said the English writer Samuel Johnson. "One should keep his friendships in constant repair."

Breakfast club

I'm one of Gloria's guys. Gloria is the head waitress at the Downtowner Coffee Shop. I used to be a pain in the rear for my wife, Dorothy. Not on purpose. It's just that after I retired from the steel company after 40 years in sales, I was home a lot and getting in my wife's hair. I wasn't a real happy camper with nothing to do and nobody to pal around with. Most of my friends were business acquaintances. Once I retired, I tried keeping in touch with a couple of them, but I guess work was the glue that had kept our friendship together.

Frank, a guy I got paired off with at the public golf course, invited me to join him and some other guys for coffee at the Downtowner. That was 4 years ago. Since then, I try to make it down there at least three times a week.

We're the regulars at the round table in the corner by the big front window where you can see the pretty girls walk by. Did I say that? Sometimes there's just three or four of us. Other times we're squeezed in tight with eight or nine around the table. Gloria serves us coffee and generous portions of grief. She says stuff like, "Why don't you bums get a job?" We all laugh and tell her we'd miss her bad coffee. We've all got mugs that say Gloria's Guys that hang on hooks near our table.

Every day we solve the world's problems, if only the world would listen. We give each other unrelenting you-know-what mostly for the fun of it, though we gave Jack some serious heat about hitting the sauce too hard. He now says we helped him stop. We were there for Bob, too, when his wife died. And we were there to help Ray figure out what to do about his wayward son. On the home front, Dorothy and I get along better because I have a life again.

Salesman — Chicago, Ill.

Points to ponder

- Seek friends and activities outside of work.
- A few good friends keep our spirits high and are tonic for daily troubles.
- Make new friends throughout your life.

Mindful connections

How do you go about building friendships? For starters, try going out of your way to meet people. If you're part of a faith community, look for opportunities to get acquainted with newcomers. Connecting with a spiritual community often provides welcome friendships, along with the mental and emotional benefits that come from reaching out to a higher power. Consider putting together a regular Friday night dinner gathering of couples who might enjoy one another's company. Make a point of introducing yourself to new co-workers, especially those whose life experience and age may be different from yours. You can also find social sustenance by joining a group that shares a common interest, such as gardening or dancing or bridge.

Make a special effort to stay in touch with your friends from childhood. These are the people who share a past with you, even if you no longer have any interests or work in common. Treat your family as friends, too, dropping them notes and keeping current on their special occasions. With the proliferation of the Internet, it's now possible to connect regularly with friends and family via e-mail — and to use message boards, chat rooms and Usenet groups to locate new companions who have mutual interests. These days there are even machines called information appliances, which provide access to the Internet and are as easy to use as a telephone.

Then there's volunteering. Studies of older adults reveal that those who willingly give to others are healthier, better adjusted and less lonely than those who don't. So far older Americans haven't tapped into this resource in large numbers. Although 70 percent of seniors currently offer some sort of informal help to friends and relatives, two out of three don't do any volunteer work. The most active volunteers contribute less than 4 hours a week.

Whether you spend your time with old friends, family members or people in need, it all boils down to creating a circle of love. Being with others, and even taking care of others, improves social integration and self-esteem — not just for you, but for everyone involved. When you take your grandchildren to the zoo or accompany your parent to the doctor, you've lightened their lives and improved your own prospects for the future, too. Likewise, when you deliver meals to poor people or help someone learn to read, you've also done your own health and well-being a favor.

Give of yourself

Volunteering can be a good way to give back to your community — and it will also benefit your own life and longevity. We all have gifts (abilities) to share. But who needs your help the most? You can find opportunities in nearly every town in America. Check the government section of your local telephone book for names and phone numbers. Also, most churches and schools will gladly accept any assistance you want to give. Consider the following examples:

Service Corps of Retired Executives (SCORE). SCORE is an organization of former corporate executives and managers who offer their services to startup entrepreneurs and other small businesses. These locally chartered volunteer organizations, funded by the Small Business Administration, provide free assistance and seminars. Every one of them needs mentors, workshop leaders and other helpers.

www.score.org
409 3rd St. S.W., 6th Floor
Washington, DC 20024
800-634-0245

Senior Corps. Senior Corps, which is affiliated with the Corporation for National Service, links more than 450,000 older Americans to volunteer opportunities in their communities. Its main programs include:

- **Foster Grandparents Program.** Volunteers in this program provide emotional support to child victims of abuse and neglect, tutor children who lag behind in reading, mentor troubled teenagers and young mothers, and care for premature infants and children who have physical disabilities and severe illnesses.

- **Retired Senior Volunteer Program (RSVP).** This program matches the personal interests and skills of older Americans with opportunities to help solve community problems. RSVP volunteers choose how and where they want to serve, making it easier for older adults to find volunteer work that appeals to them.
- **Senior Companions Program.** Volunteers reach out to older adults needing extra assistance to live independently in their own homes or communities. Senior companions provide friendship to isolated seniors, assist with simple chores and furnish transportation.

www.seniorcorps.org
Corporation for National Service
1201 New York Ave. N.W.
Washington, DC 20525
202-606-5000

Generations United. Generations United combines the efforts of more than 185 national, state and local organizations, representing more than 70 million Americans. The group promotes the mutual well-being of children, youth and older adults.

www.gu.org
122 C St. N.W., Suite 820
Washington, DC 20001
202-638-1263

Older Adult Service and Information System (OASIS). OASIS serves more than 350,000 members over age 55 in 26 U.S. cities. Volunteer opportunities include an intergenerational tutoring program, teaching classes and program management.

www.oasisnet.org
7710 Carondelet Ave.
St. Louis, MO 63105
314-862-2933

Family Friends, of the National Council on the Aging. Volunteers over age 50 provide respite for families with special needs children. Programs are located throughout the country, coordinated through 47 centers with more than 2,000 volunteers.

www.ncoa.org
National Council on the Aging
409 3rd St. S.W.
Washington, DC 20024
202-479-1200

Things change

Over time, relationships naturally evolve. As you go through life, you find yourself assuming new roles, from being an unruly adolescent who ignores curfew to driving your aging parents to meetings after dark; from tossing a baseball with your own children to allowing them to help you mow the lawn as you slow down. It's a natural shift that comes with years of experience and a melding of love and obligation.

As life expectancies began to increase dramatically in the last century, another transformation was created in the world of relationships. Families of four generations started to proliferate, giving us far more healthy and active great-grandparents than at any time in history. For the first time, countless women could gather for photos with their mothers, daughters *and* granddaughters.

But people don't stay healthy and active forever. Because science has made great progress in preventing and treating many of the diseases that shorten life but hasn't resolved as many chronic illnesses, the typical person will spend more time sick at the end of their lives than ever before. Now, instead of retiring into a life of leisure, many people in their 60s will care for elderly parents that a generation ago would not have survived so long.

If you're an average American, it's likely that you will spend more years caring for your aging parents or grandparents than you will for your children. And, believe it or not, your children will spend more years seeing to your needs than you did seeing to theirs. Think about that. This is unique in history.

The caring equation

These days, more than 22 million households actively provide some type of care for their aging relatives, a figure that has tripled in the last 10 years. But many of these households have started to enlist professional help, too. Between 1982 and 1994, the percentage of

Craving connections

The average family caregiver is a woman — so is the surviving parent. How ironic, then, that mother-daughter relationships are among the most complicated we experience.

Yet Karen Fingerman, Ph.D., author of *Aging Mothers and Their Adult Daughters: A Study of Mixed Emotions*, believes that a woman's relationship with her mother or daughter is one of her greatest resources. "You have a great relationship with someone who's invested in you," she says.

If you are a woman with a mother or daughter, here are some suggestions for making your time together memorable and for enhancing your relationship:

- Look through old photo albums and have your mother identify the people in them.
- Listen to your mother tell stories from her past. It's your history, too. Record the stories on audiotape or videotape. Once she's gone, you will never again have this opportunity.
- Tell your mother about your day, but don't complain and don't expect her to solve your problems anymore.
- Prepare an old family recipe together.
- Plant a garden.
- Take a class or join a book club together.
- Travel together.
- Create a memory jar. Write down a memory of your mother or daughter every day and put it in a container. At the end of the year, present it to the other.
- Send your mother flowers on your birthday. It's her day, too.

older people receiving only informal care (defined as unpaid care provided by family members) dropped from 74 percent to 64 percent, while the use of combined formal and informal care increased from 21 percent to 28 percent).

Part of the reason may be due to a sandwich effect, as people try to simultaneously care for both their parents and their children — often while holding down a job. The words *sandwiched caregiver* or *sandwich generation* describe people caught between the needs of very young children and aging parents. But with longer life expectancy, many people taking care of their aging parents are older themselves, with children who are either grown or in college. The sandwich is no less real, because this means you spend much of your adult life meeting everyone's needs but your own.

The average sandwiched caregiver is a woman between the ages of 45 and 55 who works full time, then spends another 18 hours caring for one of her parents, most often her mother. But the entire household can get into the helping mode: Nearly one-fourth of caregiving households provide at least 40 hours each week of unpaid, informal care to an older family member. The statistics are especially surprising in light of the geographic distance between many aging parents and their adult children.

When you consider what all this home caregiving is worth, it's surprising more resources aren't available to help families attend to their kin. About 20 percent to 30 percent of employed people care for older relatives, costing businesses between $11.4 billion and $29 billion each year, according to a survey by the Metropolitan Life Insurance Company. The U.S. Administration on Aging estimates that if the work of caregivers had to be replaced by paid home-care staff, the estimated cost would be between $45 billion and $95 billion a year.

Of course, you take care of your parents because it's the right thing to do, because you want to repay the time, energy and money they spent raising you. But there's another element to this, too: how you treat your parents in their time of need gives your children an idea about how they should someday treat you. "As we care for our parents, we teach our children to care for us," wrote Mary Bray

Pipher in her 1999 book, *Another Country: Navigating the Emotional Terrain of our Elders.* "As we see our parents age, we learn to age with courage and dignity. If the years are handled well, the old and young can help each other grow."

The realities of home care

Who cares for family and friends — and how do they do it? The National Institute on Aging's National Long-Term Care Survey revealed these facts:

- Half of all caregivers are older themselves.
- Although caring for an older person with disabilities can be physically demanding, one-third of all caregivers describe their own health as fair to poor.
- Caregivers spend an average of 20 hours a week taking care of older individuals and even more time when that person has multiple disabilities.
- Because caregiving is such an emotionally draining experience, caregivers have a high rate of depression, burnout and fatigue compared to the general population.
- Almost one-third of all caregivers balance employment and caregiving responsibilities. Of this group, two-thirds report conflicts when it comes to rearranging their job schedules, working fewer hours than normal or taking unpaid leaves of absence.

Being the caregiver

Most families don't resemble the ideal TV clan of the 1950s, with carefully pressed clothes, impeccable manners and consistently loving exchanges. But during difficult times, such as when an aging mom or dad needs care, we often find ourselves wishing we could all be a bit more like *Father Knows Best.*

The responsibility for making sure parents get to the doctor or take their medications usually falls to adult children who didn't move away. That, in turn, often generates a new, and usually more intimate, relationship with parents that distant siblings can't share. As Lillian S. Hawthorne writes in her 1998 book, *Finishing Touches,* "I was the close-by, caretaking child, while my long-distance sibling came to visit twice a year. I envied my sister's exemption from the emergencies, panic telephone calls, canceled social appointments and uneasy vacations that I experienced with our parents."

Yet Hawthorne came to realize that hers was actually the easier role. "She (my sister) was less inconvenienced, but also less needed; she was left out of my parents' problems, but she was also, largely, left out of their lives."

Whether you're a close-by sibling or a distant one, you undoubtedly will have to deal with your parents' aging process in some fashion. If you live in the same city, you may find yourself handling day-to-day caregiving chores and possibly resenting your siblings who can't, or won't, pitch in. If you've made your home far away, you may get out of the routine tasks, but you will have to manage your own guilt — and the temptation to offer unsolicited advice to a sibling or a parent who may be doing the work.

The nitty-gritty

Let's say your parents live a few miles away. They're getting older: Dad can't remember a thing, and Mom's a lifelong couch potato who's clumsy. They don't need to move in with you — yet — but they do require a growing level of assistance. How can you share the caring with your spouse, children and distant brothers and sisters?

Experts insist that this is the perfect time to delegate. Make a list of all the tasks Mom and Dad need help with, then involve family members in getting them done. Maybe your children could tackle their yardwork or cook meals for them ahead of time. Perhaps your spouse might offer to inventory their household or help them get their finances in order. Even distant siblings can assist by calling your parents every morning or evening, either to remind them to take their pills or just to check in. With phones and the Internet, it's much easier to stay connected.

Of course, if they become more incapacitated, their need for help will increase. Your physically handicapped mother may fall and break a hip, which means she's laid up in bed instead of being there to remind your father to turn off the stove or the car engine. If his forgetfulness evolves into something more serious — Alzheimer's disease, for example — Dad may start to wander unaccompanied into the streets. What then?

Coping with caregiving

If you're taking care of your aging parents, spouse or other older relative, you probably feel stretched, both in time and energy. Here are some suggestions for all caregivers:

- Take charge of your own life. Don't let your loved one's illness or disability always be your first priority.
- You're doing a difficult job. Take some quality time just for yourself.
- Accept all offers of help, then suggest specific things that can be done.
- Knowledge is power. Learn as much as possible about your loved one's condition.
- You don't have to do everything. Look for ways to promote your family member's independence. Consider adult day care or foster care for your loved one.
- Trust your instincts. Most of the time they'll steer you right.
- Grieve for your losses, then allow yourself to dream new dreams.
- Watch for signs of depression in yourself (for example, loss of appetite, unexplained crying, sleeplessness). Don't put off getting professional help when you need it.
- Seek support from other caregivers. There's strength in knowing that you're not alone.
- Exercise, sleep, watch what you eat, get regular checkups.

The day I took Dad's keys

My father bought a new black Cadillac every 3 years. It was his only extravagance. He was president of our small-town bank and was well-liked. He'd started working there at age 12 polishing spittoons. Dad was a small man, his head barely above the big steering wheel of those finned boats he drove.

Ever since I was a baby, he loved to take my mom, sister and me on Sunday drives over to Newton for lunch after church. I have pictures of Dad looking serious and proud alongside every Caddy he ever owned. There's a picture of me as a toddler in his lap behind the wheel. He smiled for that one. I learned how to drive in his '62 Seville. He let me borrow the '65 for high school prom. I got in trouble for standing on the hood and playing my clarinet while a buddy drove us slow down Front Street. (Dad never had a great sense of humor.)

After Mom died, Dad was never the same. I lived in a nearby state, so I wasn't sure if it was just depression or if not taking his diabetes medicine was part of the problem. Then he had a couple of small strokes. The doctors said they didn't do any permanent harm, but he seemed different to me. We got a call one blustery night in December from the Pratts who lived down the street from dad. He'd been walking from house to house in the cold and dark, asking neighbors if they'd seen Loretta—my mom.

On a visit home, he drove me to Newton in his '95 Brougham. We took the Interstate, which he preferred to do ever since it came through back in the late 60s. The speed limit was 70, but he was going 80. He kept drifting from one lane to another. A couple times he swerved onto the gravel shoulder. I kept looking over at him and could tell he wasn't even aware he was lane jumping and speeding.

Before I went home, I had a heart-to-heart with Dad about not driving anymore. His housekeeper, Marcia, had told me she could do any shopping for him. One of Dad's poker buddies, Wayne, volunteered to drive him wherever he wanted to go. Dad wouldn't listen. In fact he got downright hostile. So I dropped the subject and drove home. Big mistake on my part. What if he hit some kid?

We continued to get phone calls from Marcia and Dad's neighbors. Today, he backed over the Larson's trash cans. Last weekend, officer Plumber pulled Dad over for running a stop sign down by the railroad tracks. The passenger side of his car has a long scratch on it. Nobody knows how it got there, but a friend of Wayne's said there was a suspicious streak of black paint on a steel guardrail behind Weirick's Pharmacy.

I made another visit on Friday, and by Saturday afternoon, it was clear what I had to do. I vowed to myself I would muster the moxie to do it. I took Dad out to eat Sunday noon, just like we'd done all my years growing up. He insisted on driving, of course, so I suggested we eat in town instead of driving to Newton. As soon as we got back to his house and he shut off the ignition, I reached for the keys. Both our hands were on them. He knew what I was doing and tried to pull them from me. "Dad, it's time," I said. "You've got Marcia and Wayne and half the town worried about you. Please give this a try for all of us."

I expected a fight. Instead he just looked at me, or rather past me out of embarrassment, and said kind of gruffly to save face, "Take 'em, if it'll stop your nagging, but if Wayne or Marcia aren't around when I want to go somewhere, you better believe I'm driving."

"It's a deal," I said, knowing he'd never see the keys again. "Let's shake on it."

Concerned son — Marshalltown, Iowa

Points to ponder

- We are always the child to our parents, but a time comes when those caregiving roles are reversed.
- Ask your adult children what problems they see in your driving.
- Learn to graciously accept help from your adult kids and friends.
- By recognizing your limitations, you avoid tragic accidents.

If you weren't already arguing with your siblings over what Mom and Dad need, this might be the time you'd start. Children who fought over whose turn it was to wash the dishes or take out the trash may not be able to help themselves. Yet the important thing to remember is that you want to provide your parents with as much love and compassion as possible — even if you're stuck with no help from your brothers or sisters. After your parents die, you'll wonder if you did the right thing, if you did all you could do. You'll find much more comfort in being able to answer yes with certainty.

From a distance

What if you're the sibling or the daughter or son who lives in another city or state? There are ways to assist or be supportive from afar, which will help alleviate some guilt you may feel at not being there full time. For example:

Call regularly. Set aside routine times to call your mother, sister or other relative who's caring for your aging parent. Suggest tasks that you might do from a distance, such as mending or researching medical plans or looking for respite care. In addition, speak with your aging parent on a regular basis. Your caring telephone call may be some of the best medicine he or she receives.

Visit often. Make a point to get home as often as possible. If you are thinking about visiting, don't put it off. It's hard to know what's going on if you're not there to find out firsthand. Your caregiving relative, as well as your aging parent, will appreciate the help and support.

Don't immediately question the caregiver's decisions. The sibling or spouse who's doing the daily, hands-on caregiving is usually the one who's in the best position to know when the doctor needs to be consulted or how often Dad should be roused from his bed. Try not to offer opinions that may be based on limited information and will only make the caregiver angry. Listen. Don't be judgmental. But be ready to step in if you see something that's obviously wrong.

Assessing their needs

How can you know how much help to offer your parents? After all, you don't want to deliver a freezerful of casseroles if they're perfectly capable of cooking for themselves. It may help to remember that about 10 percent of all 72-year-olds need some assistance with the basic activities of daily living, such as shopping, running errands or cooking. That percentage doubles roughly every 5 years. At 77, about 20 percent need some help, while at 85, nearly half require some form of aid.

You might also want to look at it this way: Divide the routine activities of daily living into two groups, personal and nonpersonal, to assess what your parents may need. Can they handle their own nonpersonal care, such as preparing meals, shopping, paying bills, using the telephone, cleaning the house and reading? These tasks are easier for others to take over, but once you're doing a sufficient number of them, you may begin to consider your parents dependent. When they can't manage their personal needs, such as dressing,

Caregiving concerns

When the National Family Caregivers Association polled its members, it found that many were exhausted. Among some of the other information the group discovered:

Predominant caregiving emotions	
Frustration	67 percent
Compassion	37 percent
Sadness	36 percent
Anxiety	35 percent
Caregiving difficulties	
No consistent help from other family members	76 percent
Sense of isolation and lack of understanding from others	43 percent
Having the responsibility for making major life decisions for loved ones	33 percent
Loss of personal and leisure time	36 percent

bathing and feeding themselves, going to the bathroom, moving from their bed to a chair, and walking, then you probably need outside help.

As long as your parents are able to manage, studies show that it may be best to err on the side of independence. People who continue to exercise control over their own lives rank themselves as more alert, active and vigorous. You may feel impatient when your mother spends too much time sweeping the kitchen floor, but if she's able to do it, you should probably let her. On the other hand, when she's writing checks to every scam artist in town, it may be time to step in and help with her finances.

The bottom line for assessing your aging parents' needs, say experts, is to provide adequate care but to encourage as much independence as possible. Even actions that may seem small to you, such as taking their opinions seriously and listening when they talk, will help them to feel that they have some control over their lives.

Contemplating a nursing home or an assisted-living facility

There may come a time when your parents need to consider a nursing home — or you must think about one for them. If they've elected to reside in an assisted-living facility, then they've probably already faced such an eventuality. But if they're still living in the home they bought years ago, a potential change may cause untold stress. After all, transitions are difficult even when you're young and healthy. Imagine how it must feel to be forced into moving from a beloved home to an environment you dread, especially when you're trapped inside a body that's betraying you. And you may have lived in that same home for decades.

Only 5 percent of people over 65 live in nursing homes, and that percentage has been falling in the last decade. Still, each individual 65-year-old has a 43 percent chance of entering a nursing home at some point in his or her life, usually in very old age. In past generations, when there were more children than parents, when fewer women worked outside the home and family members lived closer to one another, it was easy to simply move Mom and Dad in with the extended family. Now that situation is often unrealistic.

Getting help

The following groups can help you find out more about nursing homes and assisted-living facilities in your area:

Consumer Consortium on Assisted Living. This national organization represents the needs of residents in assisted-living facilities and educates consumers, professionals and the public about assisted-living issues. Ask for "Choosing an Assisted-Living Facility, Strategies for Making the Right Decision," which includes a questionnaire.

> *www.ccal.org*
> PO Box 3375
> Arlington, VA 22203
> 703-533-8121

National Citizens' Coalition for Nursing Home Reform. This group serves as an information clearinghouse and offers nationwide referrals to people who have concerns about long-term-care facilities.

> *www.nccnhr.org*
> 1424 16th St. N.W., Suite 202
> Washington, DC 20036
> 202-332-2275

New Lifestyles. This company publishes regional directories of nursing homes, assisted-living facilities and retirement communities. Call for a free directory.

> *www.NewLifeStyles.com*
> 800-820-3013

Senior Alternatives for Living. Another publisher of regional directories of nursing homes, assisted-living residences and retirement communities. Call for a free copy; also available online.

> *www.senioralternatives.com*
> 800-350-0770

You have several ways to approach this difficult subject. Consider these suggestions:

Make it a joint decision. If possible, talk openly with your parents about their options. (It's best to do this before they have deteriorated.) Let them play an important role in the decision-making process and get their buy-in on every detail. Be sure they know you want what's best for them. If this facility isn't it, make sure they understand that you want to consider other possibilities.

Do your homework. There are plenty of ways to locate good nursing homes in your area. Before making any decisions, send for consumer literature and check out rankings. Talk to everyone you know who has faced a similar situation to find out what they know about the various alternatives.

Take a tour. Visit the nursing homes that sound most appealing to you. Try to involve your parents, if possible. Look at everything, from the individual rooms to public spaces, such as cafeterias and lounges. Ask lots of questions. Arrange for your parents to eat a meal at the nursing home — and go along. Make sure your choices are close enough to allow for frequent visits.

Be loving. Remember that this is a terribly frightening time for your parents. Talk, touch, share stories, connect. Beware of feeling guilty. It is part of the process. Psychologists say that your parents may react as any other survivor of extreme stress would, perhaps by yelling, crying or withdrawing. Don't take it personally. Instead, try to be as supportive and tender as possible.

It's your turn

You put your heart and soul into taking care of your parents, and you feel good about all your efforts. But before you know it, it's your turn. Now you need help from your children or other younger family and friends. Do you think it's going to be easy? "Many would rather pay strangers, do without help or even die than be dependent on those they love," wrote Mary Bray Pipher in *Another Country.* "They don't want to be a burden, the greatest of American crimes."

As we age, roles and relationships sustain us because we love other people — but we also benefit when other people love us. When it's time to give up some control, everyone worries about being a burden. How do we let others help us and still maintain our dignity? How do we allow ourselves to become a little more dependent on the younger generation?

Begin now. First of all, experts say to start early. Practice giving up some control in small ways when you're in your middle years so that it's not such a shock later on. For example, be open to learning something new from your children or other younger relatives. Especially as they get older, their knowledge of things you may want to know more about will expand. Let them instruct you.

Beloved friends. Treat your growing children as you would a trusted friend. Confide in them, when appropriate; accept their offers of help; be gracious when they pick up a carton of milk unasked. Once they're grown, you are no longer in a strictly parental role, shepherding a group of dependent, helpless children. Practice a give-and-take relationship that's based on trust and companionship — and encourage them to do the same with you. Be positive. Support their decisions even if you do not agree with them.

A calm spirit. Experts also say that no matter what happens, try to keep a good attitude. A sense of humor and a love for life not only help you accept assistance when you need it but also provide a good example to those who care for you. Just as your parents showed you what aging might be like, so you also can offer a small glimpse to your younger friends and family.

Just say no. But don't give up too much. As you age, it may be easier and faster for others to brush your hair, do your laundry or bring in your groceries, for example, instead of letting you do things for yourself. Stay in the driver's seat. As long as you can still manage your own life, you should. Learned helplessness can be debilitating.

The secret to long life
Of course, relationships involve much more than who's going to take care of you in your old age. They are the very essence of life.

When you're a child, you learn the fundamental truths about good and bad relationships: the joy from parents who love you, the hurt when a schoolmate betrays you. When you're a parent, you discover more about the universe and your place in it. When you have a cherished spouse, you connect with something that's bigger and better than both of you.

Although your roles and relationships will change throughout your lifetime, the fact remains that you will live longer and healthier when you surround yourself with people you care about and who reciprocate those feelings. As the 17th-century poet John Donne wrote: "No man is an island."

Remember, too, that it's through powerful and loving relationships that we can, in some ways, transcend aging altogether.

Caregiver help

Throughout the United States are many public and private agencies that can help you identify day-care facilities for seniors, as well as respite in-home and caregiver help. Contact these groups:

Administration on Aging (AOA). The Administration on Aging of the U.S. Department of Health and Human Services, works closely with a national network of aging organizations to plan, coordinate and provide home and community-based services to meet the needs of older people and their caregivers. Part of its service includes some 655 Area Agencies on Aging. Call the Eldercare Locator Service, which can find the Area Agency on Aging nearest to you, Monday through Friday 9 a.m. to 8 p.m., Eastern time. It offers a free directory of aging services in every state.

Eldercare Locator Service
National Association of Area Agencies on Aging
www.n4a.org.
927 15th St. N.W., 6th Floor
Washington, DC 20005
800-677-1116

CareGuide. A care management company that helps people at every stage of the aging process lead more comfortable, secure and independent lives. The organization has a network of care managers.

www.careguide.net
739 Bryant St.
San Francisco, CA 94107
800-777-3319

CareThere. A broad database of information about health care, finance, insurance, legal products and emotional support, specifically designed to help caregivers.

www.carethere.com
635 Clyde Ave.
Mountain View, CA 94043
888-236-3961

Easter Seals. Easter Seals provides a variety of services at 400 sites nationwide for adults (and children) with disabilities, including adult day care and in-home care. Services vary by site.

www.easter-seals.org
230 W. Monroe St., Suite 1800
Chicago, IL 60606
800-221-6827

Family Care America. This Web site offers varied resources to meet caregivers' specific, localized needs, including caregiver support, solution sharing and discussion forums.

www.familycareamerica.com
1004 N. Thompson St., Suite 205
Richmond, VA 23230

Interfaith Caregivers Alliance. With 1,300 programs throughout the country, this group offers respite support and a variety of other services through local congregations working together. Services vary by location.

www.NFIVC.org
1 W. Armour Blvd., Suite 202
Kansas City, MO 64111
816-931-5442

National Adult Day Services Association. This group, affiliated with the National Council on the Aging, can furnish information about elder care centers in your area, through a telephone call or online.

www.ncoa.org
409 3rd St. S.W.
Washington, DC 20024
202-479-1200

National Association of Professional Geriatric Care Managers. Geriatric care managers are health care professionals, most often social workers, who help families handle the problems and challenges associated with elder care. This national organization can refer you to their state chapters, which in turn can provide the names of geriatric care managers in your area.

www.caremanager.org
1604 N. Country Club Road
Tucson, AZ 85716-3102
520-881-8008

National Family Caregivers Association. This Web site includes information about caregiving, what NFCA has to offer, current projects and programs and others planned for the future. Members receive the quarterly newsletter *Take Care!* inspirational greeting cards and access to an experienced staff that provides information, referrals and caregiver support counseling.

> *www.nfcacares.org*
> 10400 Connecticut Ave., #500
> Kensington, MD 20895-3944
> 800-896-3650

Shepherd's Centers of America. This organization provides respite care, telephone visitors, in-home visitors, nursing home visitors, home health aides, support groups, adult day care and information and referrals for other services. Currently, 75 centers exist nationwide. Services vary.

> *www.shepherdcenters.org*
> 1 W. Armour Blvd., Suite 201
> Kansas City, MO 64111
> 800-547-7073

Today's Caregiver. This Web site for Today's Caregiver magazine includes topic-specific newsletters, online discussion lists and chat opportunities.

> *www.caregiver.com*
> 6365 Taft St., Suite 3006
> Hollywood, FL 33024
> 800-829-2734

Who will care for Mom?

I thought I'd always be there for Mother. For a while I was. When Alzheimer's robbed her of her ability to care for herself, I arranged home care and helped out myself. I drove her to church and to doctors' appointments and still managed to get three kids off to school. Then my husband got transferred to another state. We talked about taking Mother with us. She didn't want to go. Some days she'd assure us she'd be all right. Other days, she piled on the guilt.

As if I wasn't feeling guilty enough, things got worse. Mother's condition deteriorated. We had to put her in an assisted-living facility. But she wandered away on three occasions. Physically she was getting more frail, so we moved her to a nursing home. It was understaffed, and Mother would complain during her lucid moments, which were fewer and fewer. I was trying to care for my family and commute back and forth to visit Mother. It was awful. She passed away 18 months after moving to the nursing home.

I wish it had gone better, but I learned some things during that time. I learned that if I couldn't be there in person very often, I could do things to make it seem like I was. I knew the names of her doctors and key nursing home staff and talked with them regularly. I learned I should have asked Mother about her financial situation before all this happened. I should have researched long-term-care options way before we needed them.

I learned to take care of myself. I tried to exercise, eat right and get enough sleep. In Internet chat rooms, I learned others are struggling to care for aging parents in other cities. It helped to share stories and worries. I never stopped feeling guilty, but it helped to know I was doing all I could and that I wasn't alone.

Concerned daughter — Dallas, Texas

Points to ponder

- Aging parents sometimes need more care than a family can provide.
- Plan ahead and find a well-run facility before you need it.
- Don't forget to take care of yourself.

Your independence

- Be smart when it comes to safety.
- Everyone needs help now and then.
- Shop wisely for living accommodations.

If you're like most people, independence is the bedrock upon which you've built your life. More than virtually anything else, you treasure your personal freedom from the control of others. Aging, though, presents a significant challenge to the self-reliance that you've enjoyed from young adulthood onward. As the years advance, your body and mind continue to change in ways that will eventually affect your safety and security. It's those basic needs that must be satisfied first — even if it means sacrificing some of your independence along the way.

The order of those priorities holds some profound implications: Can you stay in the home for which you worked so many years to pay off and that you shaped to your personal tastes? Will your physical capabilities and surroundings allow you to do something as simple as opening a drawer — and keep you out of serious dangers such as fire or falling? Without making any changes to the way you live, will you someday be able to call for help, take necessary medication or get to the doctor's office for a checkup?

At present, an American man who lives to age 65 has a total average life expectancy that stretches for another 15 years. He will most likely spend 12 of those years living a completely independent life and the remaining 3 with some degree of dependency. A woman the same age has an average of 19 more years to live, and she can expect to spend 14 of them as an active, independent person.

Fortunately, your options for ensuring your own well-being grow more numerous every day. Whole industries have evolved to give older adults additional choices in their lives, while decreasing infringements on their independence.

But for independence to remain a key part of your life, you must be willing to objectively assess and accommodate whatever physical or psychological limitations you might experience. You must look for available coping options. And you must regularly find ways to adapt to the inevitable changes that aging brings.

In this chapter, you'll learn:

- How to keep your options open
- Ways to ensure your health, happiness and comfort at home and outside your house
- What sorts of tools can help you with tasks such as opening a door and combing your hair
- And what housing alternatives match your changing needs and preferences

Aging doesn't have to mean fewer choices. It does mean that you must make good use of the choices you do have in ways that maintain your welfare and your independence.

Staying safe

What's essential to staying independent? Your safety, of course. The longer you can watch out for yourself, the more personal liberty you'll enjoy. In most cases, your efforts to ensure a reasonable level of personal security are so automatic that you don't even realize you're constantly sifting information for possible threats and steering clear as danger arises. If your safety wasn't already important to you, it's unlikely you would have reached your current age. You are a survivor.

Aging, per se, doesn't call for greater amounts of safety, just a clearer focus on safe behavior. As you age, your potential vulnerability increases dramatically. You may become physically weaker than someone, say, even two-thirds your age. Your mental speed might slow, bringing a drop in your reaction time. And medications may adversely affect your sense of balance, touch, taste, smell and hearing.

There's a Catch-22 here: You must be safe to continue aging, but as you age it's more difficult to remain safe. And it's usually the simple things you need to reconsider. According to the Consumer Product Safety Commission, more than 600,000 people over age 65 are treated annually in hospital emergency rooms for injuries associated with products they live with and use every day. Similarly, falls in the home and community cause or lead to nearly 13,000 deaths among people 65 and older each year.

- So how do you do it? The answer is threefold:
- Heighten your awareness — in other words, be prepared.
- Adopt safe practices.
- When it's needed, get help in increasing your security measures.

Home, sweet home

It's ironic that the home, your safety net, your port in the storm, ranks statistically as one of the most dangerous places you can be. But you have to remember that the average residence does put you in regular contact with electricity, heat sources, water, slick surfaces, stairs and a multitude of other physical dangers.

For these reasons, it's particularly important to survey your home — be it a single-family residence, assisted-living facility or any other housing arrangement — with your own safety in mind.

Look for features or areas that can cause you to lose your balance or footing: stairs, rugs, electrical cords, spilled liquids, stepladders, shower stalls and the high wall of a bathtub.

Consider devices that cause burns or fires: Stoves, ovens, toasters, frayed electrical cords, faulty or overloaded electrical outlets and extension cords, outdated wiring, tobacco products, candles and fireplace flues. Bathrobes with long sleeves that may catch on fire also are hazardous.

Likewise, electrical shock can stem from faulty electrical cords, overburdened outlets, excessively worn power tools and appliances operating in or around water.

Check for potential sources of toxic fumes — gas ovens and stoves, water heaters, radiator boilers, clothes dryers and attached garages.

Pay particular attention to high-traffic areas that combine multiple threats such as water and electrical sources. The kitchen and bathrooms are the prime spots. Alone, each is among the most dangerous places in the home. Together, they can be lethal.

Safety from falls

One-third of people age 65 and older falls each year. About three-quarters of those spills happen at home, and only 5 percent to 10 percent are caused by "dangerous activities," such as climbing a ladder or standing on a chair.

That leaves a considerable number of falls owing to loss of balance, missteps on stairs, trips from feet snagged under electrical cords, and slips on rugs, runners and doormats. These falls often involve a significant amount of injury. It's estimated that 250,000 people break their hips in the United States each year, and the aging population is projected to drive that number to 650,000 by mid-century. Mortality rates within a year of a hip fracture are alarmingly high.

Throughout the house. Clearly, you need to watch your footing everywhere you go in your home. Solidly attached stair railings and substantial grab bars in bathrooms can help. At the same time, consider replacing or moving chairs and small tables that might tempt you to reach for them, only to give way under your full weight.

Clear pathways of all low furniture, decoration and clutter, such as footstools, ottomans, potted plants and the grandchildren's toys. You could easily trip over such items, especially in low-lighting conditions. Never leave lamp, telephone or computer power cords lying where you walk. Have your phone easily accessible, or use a cordless phone to reduce the risk of falls.

Night lights are inexpensive to buy and operate. Install them in outlets in your bathroom and hallways.

Extension cords can be especially troublesome. Cords that can safely carry electrical current to all but the shortest reaches will either be wide and flat or thick and rounded. Both types can be a problem on a carpeted surface. On hardwood or tiled floors, the rounded cords become a miniature roller that can quickly throw you off balance.

Always keep the stairs free of clutter. Examine the stairs' tread edges and surfaces, and replace any loose or slick material with firmly attached carpeting, sand-impregnated paint or other similarly sure-footed coatings. Additional lighting can also make most stairways safer.

Because of their curled edges and the often-slick nature of their weaves, throw rugs can cause particularly treacherous footing. First decide whether the traction provided by the rug is better for you than the bare floor surface underneath. If the runner lies atop carpeting and serves only as a decoration, eliminate it.

If you must use a rug in a particular area, choose one with an attached, nonslip rubber backing. To keep the rug flat and stable, consider using nonslip netting, mesh tape, underpadding or spray-on coating. Strong lighting near the rug also reduces your chances of tripping.

Kitchens and bathrooms. Bathrooms and kitchens can be nightmares of dangerous footing. The combined elements of water, soap and small items that are easily dropped provide particular challenges to older adults. Common sense and the willingness to slow down will help immensely. If you fumble or spill something, pick it up or mop it up immediately. If you put off the chore, you could soon find yourself sliding into a fall.

Stepping over a bathtub wall is enough to make many people momentarily unstable, no matter what their age. Consider adding a grab bar or a safety railing, a U-shaped device that clamps to the

Light up your life

Aging takes a natural toll on your vision. You can expect advancing years to bring a reduced ability to see fine detail, a narrower field of vision and drastically diminished sight after dark. When you are 70, your eyes will need three times longer to adjust to the dark than they did when you were 25.

Lighting is the easiest and most practical way to improve vision safety in your home. Be prepared to add more than just an extra lamp or two. At 40, most people need 145 watts of light to adequately see close work. At 60, that requirement jumps to 230 watts, and at 80, to more than 400 watts.

Start by increasing the wattage in the lamps you currently use. Be careful to stay within the manufacturer's recommended range for each fixture, which is marked on it. Add more task lighting around desks, reading chairs, workbenches and kitchen counters. Adjust work areas so that they're closer to natural light sources, such as windows and skylights.

Consider a combination of incandescent, fluorescent and halogen lighting. Fluorescent bulbs usually produce fewer shadows. Incandescents provide greater contrast, and halogen lighting is thought to come closest to sunlight. Be aware, also, that too much light used in the wrong way can produce a blinding glare.

Areas of your home that may need the greatest lighting improvement include stairways, storage closets, the garage, storage sheds, hallways, outdoor pathways and places with a change of floor heights, for example, a sunken living room or a raised dining area.

Ask an electrician about adding three- and four-way wall switches to your heavily used rooms. These allow you to control lights from more than one location, saving you a trip across a dark room. The technology for remote control switches has improved dramatically, as has the cost of these safety devices.

Finally, motion-sensitive outdoor lighting accomplishes far more than discouraging intruders from your home. The automatic lamps can make parking and trips between your car and door safer and more secure.

tub's side, for extra stability. You can also create better footing within the tub itself by adding a suction cup mat or adhesive rubberized strips.

Finally, give some thought to what to do if you fall. Moving with your momentum and rolling on a hip or a shoulder can ease your way down and save broken bones along the way. Dislocated shoulders and cracked forearms are common among those who try to arrest their falls too abruptly. Also remember to keep a telephone nearby whenever you're on a ladder or a step stool. Should you fall, you'll have a way to call for help. Remember to always think ahead if you're alone and planning a high-risk activity.

Safety from burns

Burns cause a considerable number of injuries and deaths to older adults. Of all reported deaths related to mattress and bedding fires, for instance, 42 percent were among persons age 65 or older, and an estimated 70 percent of all people who die of clothing fires are 65 or older.

Everyday items and habits spark the majority of these tragic accidents. Ovens, ranges, cooktops, space heaters, hair dryers, curling irons and even heating pads and electric blankets can produce painful burns or start fires.

Burns can be far more debilitating than the loss of physical property. Even slight burns distract your attention, and a second or third degree burn that's improperly treated could lead to serious infection. Your best bet is to adopt practices to avoid injury in the first place.

Check yourself whenever operating any cooking appliance in your kitchen. Are you reaching across lit burners where your sleeve could catch on fire? Is that potholder in contact with a gas flame? Did you turn the oven off after removing the roasted chicken?

At the kitchen sink — and at every faucet throughout the house — remember that scalding water could be only seconds away. Reset your water heater, if necessary, to limit the high temperature to 125 F or 130 F. Remember, too, that water use elsewhere in the house, be it from a flushed toilet or a running shower, can affect the water temperature delivered at other spigots. A plumber can add heat-sensitive valves to faucets or showerheads to reduce the chance of scalding.

Avoid extension cords when using small appliances, such as hair dryers and toasters. The small-gauge electrical cords common in most homes are generally inadequate for these devices.

It pays to plan

A few years ago when our youngest graduated from college, it dawned on me that we were empty nesters. Now our babies were grown, the house was paid for and my husband was entering the final years of a successful career.

Our accountant did some figuring for us and said there was no real financial advantage for my husband to stay on at the company until age 65. Early retirement appealed to him, but he wanted to keep working part time after he retired, because so many of his friends had deteriorated rapidly after they retired.

We sat at the kitchen table one night and began to plan in earnest. Do we want to keep living in our hometown? In this house? Do we want to live somewhere else just in the winter? If we moved somewhere else, would we miss home? Would we buy a house or a condo? Would we be happy living where everyone else is retired, or do we want more of a mix of people?

We are both in good health with many interests, including our enjoyment of skiing, downhill and cross-country. We also like to play golf, but neither of us likes excessive heat and humidity. Winters where we live are cold and sometimes snowy, yet winter can be a wonderful time of year. Still, if we lived where winter was a bit milder, you wouldn't hear us complaining.

We decided we would greatly miss this part of the country that had been our home since childhood — the oak forests, the green hills and all there is to love about each season. Maybe we could find a retirement community that still had seasons with all the recreational activities we enjoy.

Over a period of 5 years, we visited several communities, retirement and otherwise, in different parts of the country. We mingled with residents to get a feel for the types of people who live

Aging can affect your circulatory system, causing your extremities to become cold and numb. For that reason, it's common for older adults to rely on small, portable space heaters for supplemental warmth. These appliances can be safe, but you must use them with care. Most of these heaters are lightweight and therefore easily

there. We looked for a town that had a college because we both like to take classes. We looked into the quality of health care in each town as well as proximity to a major airport so we could visit our children and grandchildren with relative ease. The best thing we did was to rent a condo for a month in each place.

My husband interviewed at a couple of companies. We narrowed our choices to three locations. During the few years remaining before my husband retired, we rented a condo for a week or two at each location. We subscribed to the Sunday edition of the local newspapers and used the Internet to keep up with what was happening in what could be our future home.

We chose a university town in Colorado. My husband took early retirement at 62 and we moved — just like we planned. Though he could not find part-time work (he says because of his age), he volunteers his expertise with a not-for-profit arts organization. I'm getting my second bachelor's degree, this one in art history.

We have many new friends and love our new life. Everything we want is here.

Empty nester — Boulder, Colo.

Points to ponder

- The time to think about retirement is well before you retire. Take stock of your finances, your leisure interests and geographic preferences.

- Get to know potential retirement locations. Visit in different seasons. Stay for extended periods. Talk to the locals. Rent for awhile.

- Retirement can be particularly hard on a person's health. Research potential retirement careers or volunteer work. Keep yourself reasonably busy.

tipped over. Look for units with an automatic shut-off switch in case of an upset.

Small space heaters are also tripping hazards, potentially causing a burn and a fall. Place the heater out of your walking paths and, if possible, leave it in the same location — preferably a corner — so that you know where it's sitting.

Wood burning stoves and fireplaces are other potential sources of accidental fires and burns. Even if you've spent years enjoying either, remember that diminished sight and smell could allow a spark or an ember to develop into a considerable flame before you're aware of it.

Never attempt to ignite a stove or fireplace logs with lighter fluid, gasoline, paint thinner, charcoal starter or other flammable liquids. Moreover, be certain that all flammable and volatile fluids are either stored outside your home or at least away from open flames like water heater pilot lights.

Certainly if you smoke, you're aware that fires are easily started by smoldering tobacco. What you may not consider is how simple it is to fall asleep while smoking in bed or how age may slow your ability to react if you see that a fire has started.

Whether to warn of an accidental cigarette fire or a flaming skillet of grease, smoke detectors that are in working order should be in every home. These loud and sensitive alarms are particularly important if your senses are dulled by age or medication. Place at least one device on each floor of your home and additional units near bedrooms. Check your smoke detectors each fall and spring. Change batteries annually. And have an easily accessible fire extinguisher on each floor of your dwelling.

Safety from suffocation

Like home fire hazards, suffocation can affect you before you have time to react. Even if you recognize a problem, you may be too weakened to respond.

Natural gas and other fuels used for cooking and heating must be contained and controlled at all times. Forgetting to properly turn off a stove burner ranks among the easiest and most common ways that toxic gas can begin to accumulate. Make it a habit to double-check that you've completely shut off gas ranges and ovens when you finish cooking. Don't use either appliance for extra heating.

Water heaters and clothes dryers also are commonly fueled by gas. If you're unsure about your appliances, ask a service technician to look at your system. Have the same professional inspect your appliances' exhaust vents and fuel burning components on an annual basis. Each time you use your dryer, clean the lint trap, as blockages can lead to exhaust problems and cause a fire hazard.

Numerous space heaters on the market are fueled by kerosene or liquid propane (LP) gas instead of electricity. Read all of the manufacturer's material that comes with these appliances, particularly the warnings about adequate ventilation. Avoid using these devices unless you're fully aware of their potential to cause suffocation.

Fireplaces and wood burning stoves, besides increasing fire hazards, can also deliver deadly carbon monoxide. And the vapors from stored gasoline, oil-based paints and other flammable fluids have been known to cause breathing problems.

Because many homes include attached garages, you cannot overlook the potential for carbon monoxide poisoning from your car. Warming the engine on a winter day can cause exhaust to leak into the rest of the house. Numerous deaths also have been caused by older adults who drive into their garage and forget to turn off the engine before lowering the garage door.

A wide range of carbon monoxide detectors is available for home use. These can be hard-wired into place, powered by batteries or, most conveniently, plugged into wall outlets. Consider installing one on each floor and near appliances that burn gas.

Safety from electrical shock

Given the forces involved, electricity is one of the safest systems in your home. It's quite easy, however, to put yourself at risk of a mild shock or even electrocution.

Using your home's electrical system according to its design should help you avoid most dangers. Don't overload electrical outlets. Minimize the use of extension cords. If they can't be avoided, use cords with larger wire — ones with a sufficient amp or wattage rating.

Use caution around unusually warm or hot light switches and outlets. Unsafe wiring probably is causing this condition. Exposed wiring or wires with cracked insulation can present a shock hazard. Have an electrician repair all of these.

Be particularly aware of electricity in your kitchen and bathroom. In both areas it's easy to overload outlets with appliances. Even devices like mixers and hair dryers can deliver shocks if they are exposed to the wet conditions around sinks and bathtubs. Electrical outlets near indoor water sources and all outdoor outlets should be wired with ground-fault circuit interrupters (GFCIs). Ask an electrician about these very sensitive circuit breakers, which reduce your risk of electrical shock.

In the same way, be aware of larger appliances and water. If you happen to let the sink overflow while you answer the doorbell, for example, the refrigerator could be operating in standing water by the time you return. In such cases, call for help instead of risking electrical shock by handling the situation yourself.

Your world at large
Even though statistically you're more likely to have an accident at home, the outside world contains a slew of safety challenges for older adults. Whether you're walking to the neighborhood library or sightseeing in the Grand Canyon, it's important to heighten your awareness of age-related dangers. Several key areas include:

Motor vehicles. Automobile-related injuries and deaths increase dramatically among older people. The American Association of Retired Persons (AARP) estimates that nearly 25 million drivers over 65 are still on the road. Traffic accidents injure 139,000 and kill more than 7,600 older adults each year.

This means that as you age, you need to remember that your sight, energy level, hearing and reflexes may be diminished. This will affect your performance behind the wheel. If you're unsure of your driving abilities, it's best to avoid the freeways. Also avoid anything that will interfere with basic driving operations, such as a cellphone, eating, or reaching for dashboard controls. Consider buying equipment that can help your driving — such as blind spot mirrors or electronic turn signal reminders. And check with your local department of motor vehicles about refresher driving courses. Completion of a driving course may reduce your auto insurance costs.

Walking. Ranked as one of the best exercises you can do, walking still puts older adults at risk. Studies have ranked motor vehicle accidents involving pedestrians 65 and older as among the top sources of injuries in older adults. Walk only when you're fresh and alert. Stay on sidewalks and back streets. Be sure to watch for curbs and other obstructions until you're familiar with your route. Wear bright, reflective clothing when walking after dark. Select lightweight shoes with rubber soles for walking.

Travel. Many older adults have both the available time and financial resources for frequent travel. Bring home only happy memories by following these simple suggestions:

- Before you go, check for travel advisories from sources such as the Centers for Disease Control and Prevention.

- Ask your doctor for a short copy of your medical record, especially allergic reactions and current medications, and carry this with you.

- Carry backup copies of your travel documents.

- When you're on the road, stay alert to the people and situations around you.

Independent travel offers great advantages for its aficionados. If you lack confidence in your abilities to arrange and carry out major trips, sign up for a guided tour. Being on a tour can alleviate many of the headaches and dangers you might encounter on a trip, while increasing your circle of friends.

Assistive devices: Help around the house

Everyone has heard the phrase "work smarter, not harder." If you swap "live" for "work," you'll begin to understand the idea behind assistive devices. These tools for living smarter can help you with everyday tasks, such as peeling an apple or buttoning your shirt. Some are simple handle extensions that provide more leverage, while others are ergonomically designed devices backed by space-age engineering.

"Devices!" you say. "I don't want to use a bunch of crutches just to get through the day." That initial reaction is typical — even understandable. But before you blindly categorize assistive tools as a form of weakness or physical surrender, consider how many of them we already rely on to make our lives easier and more enjoyable.

It's unlikely, for example, that you hesitate before climbing into an automobile for that short drive to the grocery store. A car is an assistive device. The vehicle helps you to accomplish your goal: getting from point A to point B with greater speed and comfort.

All assistive devices play that same kind of role, to one degree or another. Whether it's something you do every day, such as combing your hair, or once in a while, like moving heavy objects around the garden, these aids can help. Gait aids, such as a cane or a walker, can let you put more energy into mobility and less into stability — you can walk farther, faster and safer.

Attitude assistance

For those who need assistive tools to cope with aging's physical changes, attitude makes a tremendous difference in how independent or dependent they eventually become.

Consider two 75-year-olds, each of whom needs a cane for extra support. The first man views the rubber-tipped stick as confirmation that his body is broken and his physical prowess destroyed. The cane might hold him up for a few more years, but then he's certain he'll be forced into a wheelchair or, worse, confined to his bed.

The second senior, though, sees his cane as a freedom staff. It's his way to guarantee stability as he moves about on his own, without seeking aid from his wife or adult son. He even shows his granddaughter how to transform the cane into a hobbyhorse, as he spins tales of horseback adventures for her delight.

Two men, similar circumstances, but vastly different attitudes about aging and living.

Attitude shapes reality.

Medical supply houses, Web sites, catalogs, your hospital's physical therapy department and even the local hardware store are full of specifically designed items and materials that can help you with daily tasks. By using these tools, you can ease pain, add comfort, increase safety, bolster confidence, enhance ability and sustain your independence.

Devices for daily needs

Assistive devices are most often used to accomplish simple daily tasks. Using the right tool can facilitate almost everything you need to do or want to do at home.

In the bathroom, alone, choices include folding shower seats, bathtub shorteners, grab bars, electrically elevated toilets, adjustable showerheads and single-lever faucets, among many others. You can buy long-handled brushes, combs and sponges. Several manufacturers now make toothbrushes and hand mirrors with foam rubber grips for an easier grasp.

In the kitchen, chances are you're already using small electric appliances. You can expand their usefulness by finding new ways to adapt them to your chores. Manufacturers of appliances sometimes include tips for alternative uses. Buy a jar opener that can be mounted under a kitchen cabinet or counter. Use a reacher with a squeeze-handle grasper — such as grocers used in the "good old days" — for easy access to higher and lower shelves.

Devices for movement and mobility

According to the Department of Health and Human Services, more than 7 million Americans use assistive devices to accommodate mobility impairments. A cane, crutches, a walker or a wheelchair can dramatically help extend or increase your independence.

These tools come in a multitude of sizes, weights and design, so it's best to have a health care professional recommend the one that would be most appropriate for you. Ask the same person to help you determine the proper size and fit, as well as the best ways to use it.

It's a common mistake, for example, to choose a cane that's too long. The extra length pushes up one arm and shoulder, causing strain to those muscles and the back. The candy-cane-style cane (one with a curved handle) probably won't be the most comfortable if you use a cane daily. Instead, one with a swan-neck handle will put your weight directly over the cane's shaft.

A bend in the river

On one of our first dates, Mary took me to her favorite spot — a shady bend in a small river outside of town. We skinny-dipped and I fell in love. Every summer since, we go back to our special spot.

For 35 years I rose through the ranks at the company to become chief engineer. Mary taught high school chemistry. We lived well, but not extravagantly, preferring the simpler pleasures of a swim in the river, time with our children and a good book by the fire. When it came time to retire, we were ready to ride off into the sunset and travel the world. Then it all fell apart.

Mary was becoming a little less sharp and a little more forgetful. She missed one of our grandchildren's birthdays, which would have been normal for me, but not Mary, the doting grandmother. A couple times, she locked herself out of the house. Then she left a burner on and set off the smoke alarm with burning food. These were not happening all at once, so we laughed about "senior moments."

It wasn't so funny when Mary set her nightgown on fire with a candle. Then she called from the mall saying she couldn't find her car. She later confessed she had been searching for a car we'd traded in years ago. Worse yet, she had taken the bus to the mall.

Our neighbor suggested Mary be evaluated. Her internist gave her some initial tests and told me it could be Alzheimer's, then again maybe not. He referred her to a specialist for more tests. They tested her memory, her blood, her spinal fluid and gave her an MRI scan. It was Alzheimer's. They gave us the soft sell: lots of good years left, help is available. But Mary understood — and so did I. We were staring into the void. Numb. Shocked. Bewildered.

Now we take it a day at a time. I help her dress in the morning and feed her breakfast. Some of it is sad and funny at the same time. For example, she doesn't want to change into pajamas at

Awkwardness with any device is natural. Remember the first time you tried riding a bike or casting a fishing rod? Ease will come with practice.

bedtime. It's as though she doesn't have a sense of day and night anymore. Time of day and day of the week are irrelevant. We struggle. Half the time I just let her sleep in day clothes if that's what makes her happy. In more lucid moments, a memory of an old friend or event surfaces. She'll try to ask me about it, but the words aren't there. It's the "long goodbye."

We had plans for Paris, the Canadian Rockies and many more exotic destinations. Now a couple hours at the mall is good enough. We're doing OK. Mary is not prone to violent outbursts like so many Alzheimer's victims. She cries sometimes and has long spells of depression, but mostly she wanders the garden, looks at photographs and sits by the den window.

Last summer, I took Mary to the river like always. I helped her ease into the warm water. We stayed shallow. A grin of enjoyment passed across her usually blank face. We lingered. I climbed out first to help her out. She took my hand, but her face wore a look of dread. She stiffened. I coaxed her ashore, knowing that we could not come back here again. It occurred to me she may have forgotten how to swim.

I don't want to be alone. I'm scared one day her body will be here, but she will have vanished. During our 40 years together, we've had good times and a few bad times. Now any time at all is good.

Electrical engineer — Rockford, Ill.

Points to ponder

- Life takes unexpected turns. Attitude adjustments may be necessary.
- The life you have is better than no life.
- Never squander time. It's all you have to spend.

Technology also offers a wide variety of assistive devices to make driving easier. For example, hand controls can be mounted on a steering column. Wheelchair loaders and van lifts improve access. The cost for more advanced equipment can be high, but the mobility they provide can be priceless.

Devices for health and fitness

Mountaineers often use ski poles while hiking rough terrain. You can do the same for a walk around your neighborhood. Or use small hand weights, which come with a variety of grips, to add resistance to your workouts. Another option is gripless wrist and ankle weights.

Stationary bicycles, stair-steppers and treadmills make great assistive additions to any home gym. They give you better stability and a way to regulate your workout routines. If you have access to a swimming pool, look at the variety of flotation equipment water-trained runners and water aerobics enthusiasts commonly use. This equipment can add to your own training program. Select devices and activities that are easy on your joints.

Devices for information gathering

"Knowledge itself is power," said Sir Francis Bacon. And, he might have added, power means independence. One of the most useful assistive devices at your disposal is the computer and the access it gives you to the Internet, the most rapidly growing communication medium in history.

If you've embraced this technology, good for you. But if you're resistant to it, you're missing out on a tool that can bring the world to your door. The Internet can transport you to just about anywhere, including the reference department of the New York Public Library or the tourism office that serves your next travel destination.

Should you want to, you can use a computer to buy gifts and have them delivered, to order groceries, to send or view family photos or simply to chat with a friend who lives across the country. The Internet's wealth of information and contacts can help you no matter what you want to accomplish, whether it be facing new medical challenges or finding a good plumber.

Consider taking a computer class as a way to get started. They're fun, and you can meet other people with the same interests.

An open mind
Assistive devices cannot do all things for all people. But it's far more common for people who are new to the equipment to marvel over how much easier life has become with that extra little bit of assistance. To maintain your independence, be objective about your physical limitations — and the tools that can help you overcome them.

Where to live

One of the chief advantages to maintaining your independence for as long as possible is being able to decide where you'll live. It's no surprise that, according to AARP surveys, nearly 90 percent of older adults say they would prefer to live and die in their own homes. Although most people fear that someday they'll be helplessly trapped in a nursing home, U.S. Census Bureau figures show that only 5 percent of Americans over 65 live in these facilities. By contrast, more than 90 percent of older adults either live in their own homes or with family members.

Staying in your present dwelling is only one of many options. Broadly speaking, your choices will fall under four categories: independent living, shared living, shared semisupported living and fully supported living arrangements. Ultimately, where you live and how much support you choose will depend on your physical and mental conditions, personal preferences, interests, financial resources, family and your willingness to adapt to change.

Independent living
Home. The word alone suggests images: the house where you grew up, your first apartment, that small bungalow you bought with your spouse, the four-bedroom where you raised your family. Home probably remains the place you feel most comfortable, safe and secure.

The right stuff

I'm lucky my mom is positive and joyful despite all she's been through. Two small strokes, osteoarthritis and macular degeneration make it hard for her to do things for herself, but she is determined to try.

An occupational therapist showed her how to use various aides and adapters. I'll never forget how pleased she was the day she showed me her new "toys." With one, she was able to pull on her support hose in the morning. With another, she could reach and grab things — her slip-on shoes and hard-to-get items in the upper and lower kitchen cabinets.

A hospital foundation helped pay to have grab bars installed in her bathtub and handrails in the hallways. We removed the carpet, so she wouldn't scuff her feet and stumble. Then we refinished the wood floors to a brilliant maple luster. We turned a back hall walk-in closet into a laundry room so she wouldn't have to use the basement stairs. We put in lots of lights, especially in the hallways.

Mom wasn't about to give up reading or doing crossword puzzles either. She discovered books-on-tape and an extensive large-print section in the library. We got her a hand-held magnifying glass with a built-in light she says is wonderful. With a couple of mouse clicks, my husband activated the large-type mode on her computer. He's been teaching her how to surf the Internet. Of course she gave up driving years ago, but she has a monthly senior bus pass. A special van for people with disabilities takes her places that are not near a bus stop.

Now she has all the right stuff, including a good attitude, to live independently.

Concerned daughter — Roanoke, Va.

Points to ponder

- Roll with the punches and stay positive. Positive people tend to live healthier and longer than pessimists.

- Many communities have an array of services to help those with disabilities keep their independence.

- Accept your limitations with dignity. Don't look back in anger.

Your existing home may be the best choice if you're contemplating or just settling into the later years of your life. Maybe you've already paid off your mortgage, so except for taxes and maintenance you're virtually home free. Perhaps you've rented an apartment for years, but it's home, and you really can't see moving out of the city.

But before you start saying, "They'll have to carry me out feet first," take an objective look at your present residence to be sure it makes sense long-term. Nearly 98 percent of all housing in the United States is designed for able-bodied occupants, despite the fact that a large portion of the population will need special housing sometime in their lives.

Will you be able to safely handle the stairs of your two-story home for years to come? Is the only bathroom on the second floor? Does the large lot still hold some appeal, or is the upkeep becoming a burden?

More than 60 percent of older adults reside in homes that are more than 20 years old. Large repairs become more common as major systems such as plumbing and heating wear out.

Regardless of your home's age, the house or apartment must accommodate your mobility level, include safety systems such as strong railings and smoke alarms, and offer sufficient lighting and doorways wide enough for a walker or a wheelchair. It should require nothing more than minimal effort for anything needing manual operation or physical exertion.

Making changes. Modification may be the key to staying in your treasured home, essentially adding years to your time there. You will have to commit to doing or having the work done.

Whether it's changing doorknobs for more easily operated lever handles, replacing the front steps with a ramp or reworking the kitchen for better access, well-thought-out remodeling plans can build new life into your home. At the same time, safety features can be dramatically improved. Research suggests that up to 50 percent of home accidents can be prevented through home modification and repair. Ask local architectural associations, local senior centers, trade groups and building material suppliers to refer you to contractors who specialize in this area.

Changing single-family homes. A cold, hard look at your house might convince you that it's time to move while you're still in good physical condition. Maybe a single-story ranch makes more sense, or maybe all you really need is a two-bedroom home. Downscaling could also ease your expenses and maintenance, whether you do it yourself or hire others to help.

If you're considering building a home for retirement or are contemplating extensive remodeling of your current home, take a closer look at "universal design." This is a relatively new concept of designing housing for the occupants' lifetime. Different from "accessible housing," which refers to homes with wider doors, ramps and other aids, universal design considers the changing

Health care at home

Health care provided in your home may be one of your best options for remaining in your present house or apartment throughout the rest of your life. The two major downsides to this plan are the cost and management. But if you have the financial resources and can handle the management of a care team yourself or entrust it to family or friends, you end up with the most independently focused aging option available.

Home care is generally divided into three types:

Skilled care is conducted under the direction of a doctor and consists of services provided by health care professionals such as nurses and therapists. It can also include activities such as home dialysis, medical social work and physical therapy.

Home support services include tasks such as housecleaning, running errands or meal preparation. These types of services may be all you need to allow you to continue living independently in your own home.

A combination of these services might involve a home-care team made up of some combination of the following: physician, social worker, registered nurse, dietitian, home-health agency, visiting nurse service, therapy specialist, home-care aide, chore worker and others. This team can carry out a detailed care plan tailored to meet your specific needs.

needs of long-term residents throughout every system, surface and use of the home. Such forethought and specialization can mean higher upfront costs, but the expense can be spread over a much longer period. For more information, see *www.design.ncsu.edu*.

Other independent options. If you choose to move, you still have many options for a simplified independent lifestyle. Standard apartments, condominiums and townhouses can all provide the living space you need without the worries of exterior upkeep. Nearby neighbors can offer both social and safety advantages as well.

Retirement communities, providing a variety of housing options within their complexes, represent another option. The best of these reduces the hassles of home ownership, draws like-minded older adults together and delivers the community services their residents most want and need. But you may miss the exposure to families and younger neighbors.

Continuing-care retirement communities or life care communities go further still. These facilities offer multiple services on an a la carte basis so that as residents' needs change, they can receive additional care within the same setting. This may be your best option if you want to make only one move, and you're convinced that the managers and owners of the facility can provide the independent living setting that you want now and the assisted-living and skilled-care settings you may someday need.

Shared living

Despite its freedom, living alone is not for everyone. You can gain some real advantages, both for your emotional well-being and your physical safety, by sharing your residence, moving in with another person or family, or finding a group of like-minded individuals to share living arrangements with.

House sharing. Sharing your home with one or more people or joining someone else in his or her home can be a joy, a disaster or something in between. Consider any arrangement on a trial basis to start, and have open discussions about rent, cooking, cleaning and personal space. Consider writing down the arrangements. Groups such as the National Shared Housing Resource Center (*www.nationalsharedhousing.org*), a nonprofit clearinghouse for shared housing information, are a good place to start.

Family connections. Moving in with family used to be the way most older adults transitioned out of their own homes. But with today's far-flung families, that's not always an option. If you want to live with your children or they're urging you to move in with them, have a frank discussion about each other's expectations. Consider everything from spousal relationships, to finances, to living space allocations, to baby-sitting and child rearing before you pack the first moving box.

Co-housing. Unrelated people often enjoy the advantages of living as a family unit. Organizers throughout the country offer a collection of privately or cooperatively owned small-group residences. These arrangements usually include a live-in manager and at least some staff, but they're primarily for residents in at least relatively good health. That means people who are able to walk unassisted and tend to their personal needs without help. For more information see *www.cohousing.org.*

Senior community. Approximately 3.5 million older Americans live in multiunit housing developments. About 20,000 of these developments are federally subsidized and built specifically for older adults. Older adults with minimal income and assets may qualify for such federally funded senior housing.

Both subsidized and private multiunit developments usually include service coordinators who can represent residents as a service broker, a community builder, an educator, an advocate and a quality assurance monitor, among other responsibilities.

Other shared living options. Two together-yet-separate options you might consider are a self-contained accessory apartment within your offspring's larger home and ECHO housing. ECHO stands for Elder Cottage Housing Opportunity and refers to a small, semi-temporary housing unit on the lot of a single-family home. This option can work well, provided lot size and zoning allow for it. For more information see *www.seniorresource.com.*

Shared semisupported living

If you expect to need some assistance with bathing, dressing, meal preparation and housekeeping, then shared, semisupported care could be a valid alternative to hiring private help in your own home.

Continuing-care retirement communities, board-and-care homes, retirement centers, congregate housing and senior residential housing all offer varying levels of support staff, depending on the operator and the residents' needs. Foster family programs, usually community run, offer similar services on a one-resident-per-host-family basis.

These assisted-living centers usually offer a menu of options, allowing you to tailor your services and costs to your specific needs. Facilities that provide fewer services usually allow outside specialists to give you private help if you need it.

Many assisted-living arrangements charge a monthly rental fee for an apartment with utilities, meals, housekeeping, laundry and an emergency call system. Additional services include extra fees.

These supervised living arrangements work well for residents who have moderate functional impairment. Lately, condition-specific facilities, for example, one that treats Alzheimer's patients, also have opened. None of these replace nursing homes, which offer fully supported care, but they are a reasonable alternative for people who require some assistance.

Fully supported living

For most older adults, nursing homes rank as the last resort. People feel that such living arrangements signal not only massive physical and mental decline but also a dramatic loss of independence. Despite such impressions, in the right circumstances fully support-ed care can be a wonderful option.

Fears that you'll end up in either an intermediate-care nursing home or a skilled-nursing facility are probably among the most unfounded in the senior population. Between 25 percent and 50 percent of people over 65 will need this type of care, and half of those people will have short-term stays. The number of viable alter-natives, described above, also means that those who traditionally might have considered fully supported care can actually thrive in an assisted-living environment instead.

If you expect to move to a nursing home someday and you want to have a say in that decision, now is the time to act. Have some candid conversations with family members or friends whom you trust to make decisions for you. Visit someone who's already in a well-run nursing facility. Create a plan that will set your mind at ease for the future.

The federal government uses publicly accessible surveys to track data on individual nursing homes. The information is often old and limited in scope, but it can give you an idea of how a facility operates. Although nursing homes are regulated, it's impossible to legislate caring, so you have to take the human element of the staff into account when choosing a nursing home.

In terms of your independence, you would undoubtedly experience some feelings of compromise should you eventually need to move to a fully supported care facility. But you still have the power to choose how you think about those challenges and how they shape your outlook on life.

And finally, keep in mind that nursing homes often have waiting lists for admission. Your name on the waiting list does not commit you, but it does give you the option of moving in once a bed opens up.

Healthy aging resources

Administration on Aging (AOA)
U.S. Department of Health and Human Services
www.aoa.gov
330 Independence Ave. S.W.
Washington, DC 20201
202-619-0724
Information on pension counseling programs can be found at *www.aoa.gov/pension.*

Alliance for Aging Research
www.livingto100.com
Calculate your life expectancy.

Alzheimer's Disease Education and Referral Center
National Institute on Aging
www.alzheimers.org
PO Box 8250
Silver Spring, MD 20907-8250
800-438-4380

American Academy of Medical Acupuncture
www.medicalacupuncture.org
4929 Wilshire Blvd., Suite 428
Los Angeles, CA 90010
323-937-5514

American Association of Retired Persons (AARP)
www.aarp.org
601 E St. N.W.
Washington, DC 20049
800-424-3410

American Board of Medical Specialties
www.abms.org
1007 Church St., Suite 404
Evanston, IL 60201-5913
847-491-9091

American Foundation for the Blind
www.afb.org
11 Penn Plaza, Suite 300
New York, NY 10001
212-502-7600

American Health Care Association
www.ahca.org
1201 L St. N.W.
Washington, DC 20005
202-842-4444

American Medical Association
www.ama-assn.org/aps/amahg.htm
This American Medical Association Web site identifies specialists. It's called AMA Physician Select.

American Savings Education Council
www.asec.org
Click on Savings Tools. Then go to the Ballpark Estimate Worksheet at this Web site to estimate how much money you'll need by the time you retire to maintain your current standard of living.

Bureau of the Public Debt
www.publicdebt.treas.gov
Customer Service Branch Bureau of the Public Debt
Parkersburg, WV 26106-2186

CareGuide
www.careguide.net
739 Bryant St.
San Francisco, CA 94107
800-777-3319
Assists caregivers of older adults with information and referrals, a network of support groups, and publications and programs that promote public awareness of the value and the needs of caregivers.

CareThere

www.carethere.com
635 Clyde Ave.
Mountain View, CA 94043
888-236-3961

This Web site offers a broad database of information about health care, finance, insurance, legal products and emotional support, specifically designed to help caregivers.

Center for Universal Design

www.design.ncsu.edu
North Carolina State University
College of Design
Box 8613
219 Oberlin Road
Raleigh, NC 27695-8613

Certified Financial Planner Board of Standards

www.cfp-board.org

Cohousing Network

www.cohousing.org
1460 Quince Ave., 102
Boulder, CO 80304
303-413-9227

Consumer Consortium on Assisted Living

www.ccal.org
PO Box 3375
Arlington, VA 22203
703-533-8121

Easter Seals

www.easter-seals.org
230 W. Monroe St., Suite 1800
Chicago, IL 60606
800-221-6827

Elder Cottage Housing Opportunity (ECHO)

www.seniorresource.com
PO Box 781
Del Mar, CA 92014-0781
877-793-7901

Eldercare Locator Service

National Association of Area Agencies on Aging
www.n4a.org
927 15th St. N.W., 6th Floor
Washington, DC 20005
800-677-1116

Contact Eldercare for a free directory of aging services in every state.

Family Care America

www.familycareamerica.com
1004 N. Thompson St., Suite 205
Richmond, VA 23230

This Web site offers varied resources to meet caregivers' specific, localized needs, including caregiver support, solution sharing and discussion forums.

Family Friends

National Council on the Aging
www.ncoa.org
409 3rd St. S.W.
Washington, DC 20024
202-479-1200

Generations United

www.gu.org
122 C St. N.W., Suite 820
Washington, DC 20001
202-638-1263

Health Care Financing Administration

www.hcfa.gov

This federal agency administers Medicare and Medicaid.

Health Insurance Association of America

www.hiaa.org
555 13th St. N.W.
Washington, DC 20004
202-824-1600

Interfaith Caregivers Alliance

www.NFIVC.org
1 W. Armour Blvd., Suite 202
Kansas City, MO 64111
816-931-5442

Mayo Clinic

www.MayoClinic.com
200 1st St. S.W.
Rochester, MN 55905
507-284-2511

Medicaid

(*See* Health Care Financing Administration;
Social Security Administration)

Medicare

www.medicare.gov
800-633-4227

> (*See also* Health Care Financing
> Administration; Social Security
> Administration)

Money (magazine)

www.money.com
PO Box 60001
Tampa, FL 33660-0001
800-633-9970

> The retirement calculator at *www.money.com*
> takes you through some basic steps to
> gauge whether the money you're putting
> away now will support you during retire-
> ment. The calculations factor in variables
> such as goals, inflation and annual returns
> on investments.

National Adult Day Services Association

National Council on the Aging
www.ncoa.org
409 3rd St. S.W.
Washington, DC 20024
202-479-1200

> This group can furnish information about
> elder care centers in your area.

National Association of Professional Geriatric Care Managers

www.caremanager.org
1604 N. Country Club Road
Tucson, AZ 85716-3102
520-881-8008

National Center for Complementary and Alternative Medicine

National Institutes of Health
www.nccam.nih.gov
PO Box 8218
Silver Spring, MD 20907-8218
888-644-6226

National Citizens' Coalition for Nursing Home Reform

www.nccnhr.org
1424 16th St. N.W., Suite 202
Washington, DC 20036
202-332-2275

National Family Caregivers Association

www.nfcacares.org
10400 Connecticut Ave., #500
Kensington, MD 20895-3944
800-896-3650

National Resource and Policy Center on Housing and Long Term Care

www.aoa.gov/Housing/SharedHousing.html

National Shared Housing Resource Center

www.nationalsharedhousing.org

New Lifestyles

www.NewLifeStyles.com
800-820-3013

> Call for a free directory of nursing homes,
> assisted-living facilities and retirement
> communities.

Older Adult Service and Information System (OASIS)

www.oasisnet.org
7710 Carondelet Ave.
St. Louis, MO 63105
314-862-2933

Organ and Tissue Donation Initiative

Health Resources and Services Administration (HRSA)

www.organdonor.gov

For a donor card, contact this government Web site.

Partnership for caring

www.choices.org

1035 30th St. N.W.
Washington, DC 20007
800-989-9455

View and download state-specific forms on advance directives, including power of attorney forms.

Pension Benefit Guaranty Corp.

www.pbgc.gov

1200 K St. N.W.
Washington, DC 20005-4026
800-400-7242

Senior Alternatives for Living

www.senioralternatives.com

800-350-0770

Call for a free directory of nursing homes, assisted-living facilities and retirement communities. This directory is also available online.

Senior Corps

Corporation for National Service (CNS)

www.seniorcorps.org

1201 New York Ave. N.W.
Washington, DC 20525
202-606-5000

This Web site will link you to the following programs in your state:

- Foster Grandparents Program
- Retired Senior Volunteer Program
- Senior Companion Program

SeniorNet

www.seniornet.org

121 2nd St., 7th Floor
San Francisco, CA 94105
415-495-4990

Service Corps of Retired Executives (SCORE)

www.score.org

409 3rd St. S.W., 6th Floor
Washington, DC 20024
800-634-0245

Shepherd's Centers of America

www.shepherdcenters.org

1 W. Armour Blvd., Suite 201
Kansas City, MO 64111
800-547-7073

Social Security Administration

www.ssa.gov

Office of Public Inquiries
6401 Security Blvd.,
Room 4-C-5 Annex
Baltimore, MD 21235-6401
800-772-1213

Today's Caregiver

(magazine)

www.caregiver.com

6365 Taft St., Suite 3006
Hollywood, FL 33024
800-829-2734

The Web site for *Today's Caregiver* magazine includes topic-specific newsletters, online discussion lists and chat opportunities.

United Seniors Health Council (USHC)

www.unitedseniorshealth.org

409 3rd St. S.W., Suite 200
Washington, DC 20024
202-479-6973

Index

MAYO CLINIC ON HEALTH

Arthritis

Chronic Pain

Depression

Digestive Health

Healthy Aging

Healthy Weight

High Blood Pressure

Managing Diabetes

Prostate Health

Vision and Eye Health

612.68   Creagan, Edward T.
MAY   Mayo Clinic on
             healthy aging

DATE DUE